Comments on **Motor Neurone Di**
fingertips' guide *from readers*

'This book will be a very useful tool for anyone diagnosed with
or affected by MND. It is set out in manageable chapters so that
people can pick it up and read what they want when they want.
In addition, the question and answer style brings to life the
issues people are facing in an easy to read format.'

Heidi Macleod,
Motor Neurone Disease Association

'I very much enjoyed reading this book and think it will be well
accepted among the many families trying to find information on
motor neurone disease.'

Sandra Wilson, Information Officer
Scottish Motor Neurone Disease Association

MOTOR NEURONE DISEASE

The 'at your fingertips' guide

Dr Stuart Neilson BSc, PhD
*Lecturer, Department of Epidemiology and Public Health at
University College Cork, Eire; Former Director of Medical
Information Systems at the Centre for the Study of Health,
Sickness and Disablement [CSHSD], Brunel University*

Dr Frank Clifford Rose FRCP
*Consultant Neurologist, London Neurological Centre, Harley Street,
London; Previously Director of Academic Unit of Neuroscience,
Charing Cross and Westminster (now Imperial College) School
of Medicine, University of London; Former Medical Patron,
Motor Neurone Disease Association*

CLASS PUBLISHING • LONDON

Printing history
First published 2003

The authors and publishers welcome feedback from the users of this book. Please contact the publishers.

Class Publishing, Barb House, Barb Mews, London, W6 7PA, UK
Telephone: 020 7371 2119 [International +4420]
Fax: 020 7371 2878
Email: post@class.co.uk
Visit our website – www.class.co.uk

The information presented in this book is accurate and current to the best of the authors' knowledge. The authors and publisher, however, make no guarantee as to, and assume no responsibility for, the correctness, sufficiency or completeness of such information or recommendation. The reader is advised to consult a doctor regarding all aspects of individual health care.

A CIP catalogue record for this book is available from the British Library

ISBN 1 85959 047 0

Edited by Michèle Clarke

Typeset by Martin Bristow

Illustrations by David Woodroffe

Cartoons by Jane Taylor

Indexed by Val Elliston

Printed and bound in Finland by WS Bookwell, Juva

Contents

Foreword

by GEORGE LEVVY

Chief Executive of the Motor Neurone Disease Association

Motor Neurone Disease (MND) is considered to be rare, yet every day in the UK at least three people are diagnosed with the disease and three people die from it.

It is a condition that undoubtedly alters people's lives beyond recognition: the lives of people with the disease, and the lives of their relatives, friends and carers.

MND is never the same for two individuals, or for those caring for them. Nonetheless, there is much to be learned and much help to be gained from sharing experiences and learning about the disease and its likely progression.

Accurate information plays a key role in helping people to understand MND, and is essential in order that they can begin to realize what is facing them and to know that they are not alone.

Publications such as *Motor Neurone Disease – the 'at your fingertips' guide* help to provide such information in a well-informed, easy-to-follow format. While such information will not alter the course of a person's MND, it will hopefully help them and their loved ones to come to terms with the future.

This book has much to offer anyone affected by MND, whether personally or professionally, and I hope it will be read not only by people living with MND, but by health and social care professionals who work in the field.

Foreword

When I was first diagnosed with MND I really needed a source of information. What a shame because this book would have been my answer. The book is a mine of information for anybody in contact with MND. Because the disease takes so many forms and progresses in so many different ways, there is no single answer to any question. The book provides lots of answers to lots of questions.

Some words of advice from me. Never be a victim of, or a sufferer with, MND, but always a fighter. A smile goes a long way on a bad day: it exercises the face and lightens everybody's life. Listen to advice from any professionals you can find, but use your imagination and your own invention to solve problems. When investing large amounts of money in equipment, plan for the worst – it saves money in the long run. For example, don't buy a stairlift unless you're sure that you won't ever, ever need a through-floor lift.

Use the Contents list, appendices and index for this book for direct access to what you need to know – some of the information hopefully you will never need. Keep the book handy because the answer may be at your fingertips.

Preface

by Dr FRANK CLIFFORD ROSE FRCP

*Consultant Neurologist, London Neurological Centre, Harley Street,
London; Previously Director of Academic Unit of Neuroscience,
Charing Cross and Westminster (now Imperial College) School
of Medicine, University of London; Former Medical Patron,
Motor Neurone Disease Association*

The target audience of this book is the patient with motor neurone
disease (MND). Just as important are relatives, friends and others
who come into contact, whether at the workplace or elsewhere.
The over-riding necessity for this publication is that, although
there are many treatments, there is as yet no cure. This state of
affairs with other diseases, it is fortunate to relate, is steadily
becoming rarer – even the two commonest causes of death,
cancer and heart disease, have many remedies. These latter two
conditions are well-known to the general public, but this is not the
case with MND and the following pages will attempt to explain the
reasons for this.

To the doctor, MND is taught to him from the earliest days of
walking the wards and the reason for this is not because it is a
common condition, but because, sad to say, it is a 'good teaching
case'; patients develop a multiplicity of physical signs which the
student must learn to detect and deduce the cause. This is how
the disorder initially impinged on my consciousness and I still
have the detailed notes of my first case over a half-century ago.

During my years of training to become a neurologist, one of my
research projects was the 'intravital staining with methylene blue
of motor end plates in MND'. This grand sounding title meant
using a recently introduced (in the 1950s) technique to show the
connections between nerve and muscle; although informative, it

gave no clue as to the cause of the disease, a mystery that still pertains to this day, in spite of countless research approaches.

As a neurologist, I had great difficulty in explaining to patients the implications of the condition but learned, on professional visits to the United States, of groups of patients with the disease and their relatives who came together to discuss their mutual problems and collect money for research. I tried to do the same in London and, although initially there was encouragement, when the disease had run its course, the interest of relatives soon waned. By a chain of circumstances, the Motor Neurone Disease Association eventually came into existence and I spoke at the first meeting in London and became its Medical Patron.

Also, in the 1970s, I was asked by the Medical Society of London to arrange a symposium for the Mansell Bequest for the furtherance of neurological studies. Because Dr Mansell had died from MND, it was an obvious choice as a topic for the first symposium. I could find only a dozen neuroscientists to participate but only a few of their topics were directly concerned with MND – a disheartening reflection of the lack of interest then displayed. The proceedings were published as a monograph entitled *Motor Neurone Disease* and was the first of its kind in the UK.

Since that time, an increasing amount of research has occurred and some of the conclusions are reported in this book. No one can guarantee a cure in the immediate future but there is now at least a drug that delays the usually inexorable progress of the disease. There is little doubt that, with increasing research and interest, the happy arrival of a cure will eventually become a reality.

Spring 2003

Acknowledgements

Our thanks go to Heidi Macleod and Gayle Sweet of the Motor Neurone Disease Association, and to Sandra Wilson of the Scottish Motor Neurone Disease Association for generously giving of their time reading through the manuscript and offering valued comments. Sandra Wilson also kindly supplied much of the data for Appendix 1. We should also like to thank Lin Newman who appears on the cover with her carers Beryl Perman and Barbara Else.

The '10 Commandments', which are given in boxes throughout the text, are dedicated to Forbes Norris, an American neurologist from San Francisco, who saw MND patients for most of his professional life and wrote several articles and books, one with Dr Clifford Rose, on all aspects of the disease.

Note to reader

There is a glossary at the end of this book to help you with any words that may be unfamiliar to you. If you are looking for particular topics, you can use either the detailed list of Contents on pages v–vii or the Index, which starts on page 182.

MND explained

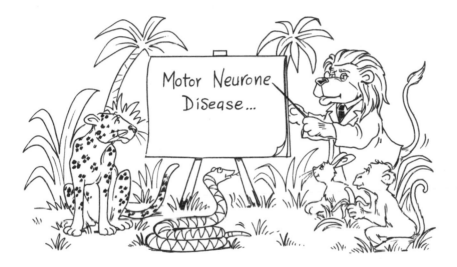

Motor neurone disease (MND) is a progressive disorder of the nervous system. Its effects on the body can be so severe that it eventually changes the lives of those affected and hence those of their families, friends and work colleagues. It is very important that the lay person understands, in simple terms, what MND is and how its symptoms show themselves. The name includes a wide variety of conditions, and so in this chapter we also discuss the different types of MND and their many medical names.

What is MND?

The term motor neurone disease (MND) covers a group of related diseases that affects both nerves and muscles because there is damage to the nerve cells that control muscle activity. Every organ in the body, such as the heart, liver, kidney, is made up of microscopic units called cells, and the nervous system is no exception. 'Neurone' is simply the medical term for a cell in the nervous system. A motor neurone is concerned with motion or movement, and motor neurones are those nerve cells responsible for moving our muscles. These are the cells that are affected in MND.

As the nerves deteriorate, signals from the brain passed by them become too weak to make the muscle fibres contract, so fewer fibres react to the contraction signals. This nerve 'degeneration' directly causes muscular weakness, because control of the affected limbs is lost. After a period of time, the muscles become weaker and thinner (wasting). This combination of weakness and muscle wasting leads to more severe symptoms resulting in poor mobility.

The nerve degeneration itself at present is not thought to be reversible (see Chapter 15 for research possibilities in this area), but treatment can slow deterioration and help maintain muscle strength, which will reduce the impact of MND on activity (Figure 1.1).

What does MND actually do to you?

The effects of MND are due to damage to the upper motor neurones (nerve cells) going from the brain to the spinal cord, and the lower motor neurones going from the spinal cord to the muscles. The nerves branch off the spinal cord to activate different muscle groups. If there is damage in the sacral region, for example, it can lead to weakness in the ankles and feet, with resultant foot-drop. By contrast, damage in the cervical region can lead to weakness in the upper body, arms and hands, all of which are directly activated by cervical (neck) nerves, as well as

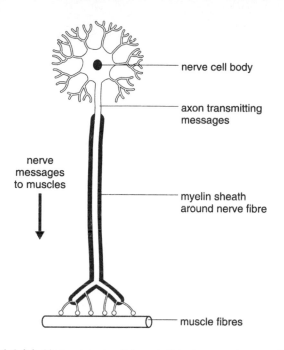

nerve cell body

axon transmitting
messages

nerve
messages
to muscles

myelin sheath
around nerve fibre

muscle fibres

Figure 1.1 (a) Normal nerve (*above*); **(b)** damaged nerve (*below*).

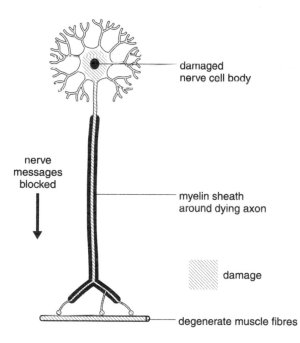

damaged
nerve cell body

nerve
messages
blocked

myelin sheath
around dying axon

damage

degenerate muscle fibres

symptoms anywhere further down. In other words, damage at this high level can also affect feet because sacral nerves receive their signals through the cervical spinal cord. This damage weakens nerve signals sent from the brain to muscles, preventing voluntary movement and, ultimately, automatic movements such as breathing. Although nerves can be damaged by injury, inflammation, radiation and toxins, it is not clear how any of these factors relate to the onset of MND. As MND progresses, motor neurones die, the affected muscles therefore stop working and people with MND become less mobile.

This loss of movement is accompanied by loss of muscle mass (called wasting or atrophy).

The brain's higher functions (thought, memory, planning, decision-making and perception), all of which can be severely affected by other neurological conditions such as Alzheimer's, are not usually involved, so the ability to think, remember, calculate etc. is not affected. It is only muscle function that is eventually lost and this may sometimes include those muscles controlling speech, swallowing and the ability to breathe.

Who gets MND?

Are there particular people who are at greater risk of developing MND?

There is no definitive identifiable group at risk of developing MND, although it is more often diagnosed in people of European descent. MND is most frequently found in the second half of life, especially those in the age group of 50–80 years. Whilst the diagnosis can be made in the late teens or young adulthood, only 10% of all new cases of MND occur under the age of 50 years; the most frequent age for diagnosis is closer to 70 years, 50% being diagnosed when over the age of 70. Both women and men can develop it but, because women in general tend to live longer than men, there are more women in this older age group where MND is typically diagnosed.

**I have heard that Britain has a higher MND population
than elsewhere. Is this true?**

The incidence (the number of people newly diagnosed each year
as a percentage of the population) and prevalence (the total percentage of the population with MND) are both higher in Britain
than anywhere in Africa or most of Asia, but the levels are similar
to those seen in the population in countries with similar age distri-
butions. Since MND develops most frequently over the age of 50,
the proportion of people in that age group in the population is the
most important factor determining the overall rate. MND is more
common in Japan, for instance, where life expectancy exceeds
that in Britain. The incidence of MND rises as the proportion of
older people in the population grows, so MND continues to
become a more significant cause of disability and death.

There are some small regions of the world with particularly
high rates of MND, and these include the Kii Peninsula of Japan
and the American Trust Territory island of Guam in the Pacific.
These two high incidence places were thought to result from
highly localized environmental effects – metal poisoning in the
Kii Peninsula and cycad toxicity in the diet of Guamanians.
Although research into these two groups provided important
insights into the possible causes of the condition (see Chapter 2),
neither hypothesis has been confirmed.

**Is MND a new disease, or has it always existed in some
form?**

MND was first described in the latter half of the nineteenth cen-
tury by the French neurologist Jean-Marie Charcot (after whom
the disease was named), but it is clear that his first description
was of a condition that already existed. At the time of this first
description, most illnesses that were not 'acute' (i.e. occurring
with a rapid onset) would have been seen as 'natural' conditions
related to age, so that MND was regarded as one of many forms of
progressive paralysis related to getting old. Whilst MND is not a
'new' disease, it is assuming increasing importance as so many
people are living longer to the ages where MND occurs.

I'm a community nurse and see more and more people with MND. Do you think that there are more cases diagnosed nowadays?

There is no evidence that MND is becoming more frequent as a consequence of modern lifestyles. Improvements in living standards, increased knowledge of diseases, and a general increase in life expectancy have led to at least a third more people being diagnosed with MND, because previously people died at ages too young to have developed MND. Improvements in diagnostic techniques and medical technology have also undoubtedly played a large part in increasing the rate at which MND is correctly identified, and accounts for a part of the increase in MND in recent decades. The incidence of MND in Britain has doubled over the past three decades and probably a third of this increase is due to improved diagnosis.

How many people in Britain get MND?

Since 1300 new cases of MND are diagnosed each year in Britain, in a population of 60 million, this means that about 4 people are newly diagnosed every day. Although accurate figures for the number of people with MND are not available for the nation as a whole, it is estimated that there are between 3600 and 7200 people with the condition, which is between 6 and 12 people in every million. Despite its comparative rarity, MND still accounts for 1 in every 500 deaths in Britain and a significant proportion of all 'chronic' (long-lasting) illness and disability.

Other names for MND

When I emailed my relatives in America to tell them about my mother's illness, they kept calling it Lou Gehrig's disease. Why?

Lou Gehrig was one of American baseball's greatest players of all time, playing 14 full seasons for the New York Yankees from June 1925 to May 1939. During his Yankees career, he played in 2130 regular-season games, was named the American League's most valuable player twice, and his team won seven World Series Championships. Lou Gehrig died in 1941 from MND, at the height of his career, aged just 38. In America he is remembered for his great sporting achievements but also the speed of his disease deterioration.

My cousin in Paris has been diagnosed with 'la maladie de Charcot'. Is this the same thing as MND?

Jean-Marie Charcot, as mentioned before, became the first neurologist to describe MND as a particular type of amyotrophic lateral sclerosis (ALS – see next section) in an extended French family. MND, in all its forms, is called 'la maladie de Charcot' (Charcot's disease) in France, although Charcot's disease amongst English-speaking doctors may sometimes be considered the name for familial ALS rather than encompassing all types of MND.

There is another disease that includes his name, Charcot–Marie–Tooth disease, which is an entirely different disease, being an inherited form of nervous system degeneration with muscle wasting restricted to the lower part of the legs and arms. This disease develops much earlier in life, is associated with loss of sensation and, despite its progressive course, causes only limited disability.

For most purposes 'MND' refers to all forms of MND in Britain whereas ALS is the broad term in the United States. The disease in Britain can be spelled motoneuron disease, motor neurone disease or motor neuron disease, which are different spellings of the same name. In this book, to maintain consistency, it will be called motor neurone disease (MND). Since these terms can be very confusing to anybody developing the disease, we explain the different types below.

Types of MND

In Britain, amyotrophic lateral sclerosis (ALS) is the most frequent distinct type of MND. ALS can be further divided into a *familial* form (where the condition is inherited) and a *sporadic* form (where it is not inherited). Sporadic ALS is by far the most common form of MND, accounting for about 90% of all people with the condition. Progressive muscular atrophy, which affects only the lower motor neurones, is a less common form of MND, and causes deterioration more slowly.

Bulbar palsy is another form of MND, but this affects speech and swallowing. The nerve cells affected are located towards the back of the brain (the brain stem). These nerve cells are a specialized group that controls the cranial nerves to the muscles related to speech and swallowing.

What is the difference between 'upper' and 'lower' MND? My neurologist mentioned it as if it was very important.

The important distinction is in the signs of the disease as revealed by the medical examination. This depends on whether the upper or lower motor neurones are mostly degenerated. Upper motor neurones are nerve cells that connect the brain to the spinal cord, extending downwards (in a collection of nerve fibres called the pyramidal tract); only a small number of upper motor neurones control many muscle fibres. Lower motor neurones connect the spinal cord to each individual muscle in the body so there are a much larger number of these. These two main types of nerve cells (neurones) are called 'motor' because they deal with movement of the muscles. The upper motor neurone meets the lower motor neurone in the front of the central part of the spinal cord (known as the anterior horn cell region).

Damage to a motor neurone will affect the muscles that it supplies with nerve impulses and possibly other nerves and muscles supplied further down the central nervous system (the brain and spinal cord). Therefore damage to a lumbar nerve might affect the lower limbs but could not affect muscles above this area. In contrast, damage to an upper motor neurone (in the spinal cord or brain) may affect muscle groups in the head and arms as well as legs.

My brother's son has had the diagnosis of MND, although he is only 6 years old. I thought it was found only in older people?

There are two conditions that affect children and adolescents that are comparable but not the same as MND in adults.

The first is Werdnig–Hoffman disease, which is usually diagnosed at birth or within the first few months of life. Also called progressive spinal muscular atrophy, it usually results in death within the first few years of life. It affects about 1 in every 20,000 children born in the UK and accounts for 0.2% of all cases of motor neurone diseases.

The second is the very rare Kugelberg–Welander disease, also called chronic benign spinal muscular atrophy, which usually affects older children or adolescents. The outlook is one of slow (chronic) progression of muscle weakness with sometimes only limited disability. Kugelberg–Welander disease affects about half as many children as does Werdnig–Hoffman disease and accounts for about 0.1% of all cases of motor neurone diseases.

Symptoms of MND

I have had a lot of weakness recently, and will be going soon to have tests to see if I have MND. Is this a significant symptom? Are there others?

The first symptoms of MND indicating that something is wrong vary from the trivial to the severe. These symptoms can include foot-drop, where the lower leg muscles fail to lift the foot when walking (resulting in slapping the foot down with consequent trips and falls), difficulty in handling small objects and dropping things, slurred speech, extreme muscle tiredness, cramps and muscle twitches ('fasciculations'), and emotional instability ('lability'), a symptom of uncontrollable laughter and crying without any obvious reason.

At the onset of MND, about 50% of sufferers will experience weakness of their arms, 25% weakness in legs or feet, while the rest have symptoms involving speech or swallowing.

Unlike many other neurological diagnoses, the mind, senses and bladder function are rarely affected in MND. This means that symptoms involving memory, thought processes (such as forget-fulness or confusion) or the senses (vision, smell, taste, hearing and touch) would be due to another disease.

Irrespective of the initial symptoms, MND will over time usu-ally affect other limbs as well. The onset can be succeeded rapidly by further symptoms, so that many have quite significant impairments by the time they are diagnosed with MND; it is always important to have an assessment as early as possible after the condition is first considered.The box opposite indicates com-mon and less common symptoms that can be expected – they are also common in lots of other conditions as well!

You talked about upper and lower MND earlier. What are the differences in symptoms?

The symptoms of upper motor neurone degeneration include stiffness (spasticity); this is assessed by resistance to passive movement (increased 'tone'). The tendon jerks assessed with a reflex hammer are exaggerated because the muscle contracts too strongly on testing. There is also widely spread, rather than localized, weakness. Because of the small number of upper motor neurones and because each upper motor neurone supplies signals to so many lower motor neurones, the symptoms are more noticeable because they will be more wide ranging.

The symptoms of lower motor neurone loss include marked weakness in individual muscles, causing partial or total paralysis with thinning of the muscles ('wasting'). In these cases there is a decrease in, or absence of, muscle reflexes as the muscles fail to contract on testing with a reflex hammer. There are also irregular and involuntary contractions ('fasciculations'). Lower motor

---

Common symptoms
- weakness
- tiredness
- depression, anxiety and insomnia
- constipation

Less common
- hunger pangs
- urinary symptoms
- pressure sores
- diarrhoea

---

neurone signs are generally more localized, affecting single muscles, although groups of muscles can also be affected.

Because lower motor neurones supply nervous impulses to a single muscle, or even a part of a muscle (in combination with other nerves signalling the rest of the same muscle), damage to a single lower motor neurone may be very limited or even imperceptible. In contrast, the effect of damage to upper motor neurones is more significant and widespread. Distinguishing between upper and lower signs can be difficult, as the initial symptoms such as weakness can be identical and both types of signs can be present; it is only by repeated assessment of symptoms that the degree of upper and lower motor neurone degeneration can be estimated.

When I look closely I can see little ripples in my muscles and I get this terrible 'creepy' sensation as if something is walking up and down my leg. If this is caused by my MND, is it going to get worse? Can I do anything to stop it?

The sensations you are experiencing are called 'fasciculations', irregular and involuntary contractions of your muscles. Because they are not voluntary but spontaneous and happening all by themselves, they can be a disturbing experience, in the same way as finding that your arm or foot in bed has 'gone to sleep' and doesn't feel as if it's part of you. Some degree of this (usually occasional and slight) is fairly common in absolutely normal people and they do not indicate anything untoward. These contractions are harmless and painless but they can be extremely disturbing. When severe or continuous, they can be a sign of damage to the lower motor neurones.

In MND, fasciculations can become more frequent and noticeable but they do not cause pain or interfere with activity but may lessen when muscle wasting occurs.

If there is pain and difficulty in mobility, they can be helped by treatment. Stiffness and fasciculations can be helped to a greater or lesser degree with the muscle relaxants baclofen (Lioresal) or dantrolene (Dantrium); cramps can be lessened using the anti-malarial treatment quinine (the chemical that gives tonic water its distinct bitter flavour), the anti-anxiety drug diazepam (Valium), or the anti-epileptic drug phenytoin (Epanutin).

As MND is a neurological disease, is it going to affect my mental capacity eventually? How soon will it start to affect my mind?

MND directly affects only the motor neurones (the nerve cells concerned with movement) – so it is unlikely that intellectual function will be noticeably affected. Many neurological conditions do have side effects of impaired thinking skills ('cognition'), confusion or forgetfulness (impairment of short- or long-term memory); research has shown that those people with MND rarely have cognitive problems that are directly related.

Those with MND have psychiatric conditions such as depression, panic attacks and other problems in common with the population at large; as the disease progresses, these may become more frequent as a response to this deterioration.

My neurologist has said that my 'mind may be spared' in MND, but my occupational therapist has warned me about emotional problems – who is right?

Strangely enough, both are correct. It is commonly said of MND that the senses (sight, touch, hearing, smell and taste) and brain function are spared – which is what your neurologist has told you. There are no psychiatric disturbances, mental illness or other mental problems associated with MND, so the severe forgetfulness or confusion that might be associated with other brain diseases are unlikely to affect people with MND.

Some people with MND find that they occasionally have emotional instability ('lability') when they laugh or cry for no apparent reason, or there is inappropriate or exaggerated emotional responses to situations, when they are unable to control these extreme feelings; this may be what the occupational therapist has warned against. Not all those with MND will experience emotional instability, since it occurs only in those who have upper motor neurone degeneration on both sides of the brain (see the next question on 'pseudo-bulbar palsy').

Depression and emotional lability must be clearly distinguished. Depression affects 30% of all adults at some time and should be treated in MND just as it should be in those without MND, with appropriate counselling and drug treatment. Emotional lability, in contrast, is a symptom associated with upper motor neurone degeneration but may be helped by medication.

My husband has been diagnosed with bulbar palsy. What sort of symptoms would he expect to have with this?

In about a quarter of all people with MND, the first symptoms at onset and diagnosis are 'bulbar' symptoms (the bulb being the hind brain) – these symptoms include slurred speech ('dysarthria') and difficulty in controlling swallowing ('dysphagia'). Bulbar symptoms are not specific to MND and are more common in those who have had strokes on both sides of the brain.

There are in fact two types of bulbar palsy depending on whether the upper or lower motor neurones are affected on both sides of the brain. Both types give difficulty in speech and swallowing but when the lower motor neurones are affected, the tongue will show thinning ('wasting') and fasciculation (called 'fibrillation') in the tongue; this type is called 'chronic bulbar palsy'. Only in the upper neurone type is there emotional lability and this type is called 'pseudo-bulbar palsy'.

The overwhelming sensation I have is lack of strength; everything is such an effort. Why are my muscles so weak?

Even in healthy people, when muscles are not used to their full capacity, the body stops using nutrients to maintain their size and volume. After some time, the muscles begin to lose mass ('atrophy') and become smaller and thinner. This wasting is much worse in MND.

Strength and muscle mass can be helped by correct diet and physiotherapy, but a full physical assessment is needed for a detailed plan, depending on the cause.

2
The possible causes of MND

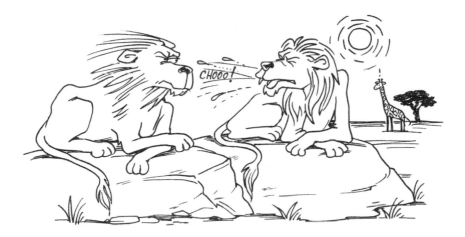

Although a great deal is known about what happens inside the body of someone with MND (the 'pathology' of MND), the cause is not known. A great many theories have been proposed, from associations with other diseases to environmental toxins, but there is no known cause that could explain all cases of MND or the distribution of MND worldwide.

In a later section we talk about genetic research in MND, the significance of having relatives with MND and its possible consequences, both for those with MND and their relatives.

Because MND is similar in its symptoms to other diseases with known causes (such as post-polio syndrome), this has led to theories about the cause of MND, but these fail to explain the vast majority of cases, even though they can explain some short-term or local effects.

One popular theory of the cause of MND was that there are differences in 'susceptibility' to MND (genetic 'predisposition') and there are external factors (such as toxins) that accelerate the disease process. The nature of the predisposition cannot be based on simple inheritance since most cases of MND are 'sporadic' and do not run in families.

Connections with other diseases

I've read in the paper that MND is caused by measles or measles inoculations. I had measles as a child – could this have caused my MND?

No. Although there have been some tentative associations reported in the past, there is no known association between any inoculation or childhood disease that withstands scientific scrutiny.

My uncle had polio and the symptoms are very like those my partner has, who was recently diagnosed with MND. Is there a connection?

There is a condition that occurs after poliomyelitis called 'post-polio syndrome' in which symptoms very similar to MND are experienced late in life, many years after exposure to the polio virus. The exposure may not even have led to disease at the time, only to what is called 'subclinical polio' where the infection is so slight that it was unnoticed at the time. It seems that damage to the motor neurones at the time of infection reduced the body's ability to cope with the normal deterioration of ageing, and motor symptoms appear in later life as a result. MND can be mistaken for post-polio syndrome because the two conditions have some similar features.

Environmental connections

I'm of West Indian descent and have had MND for 3 years, but everyone else I know with MND is white. Am I unusual in this respect?

MND is certainly less frequent in Asia and Africa, and in Asian and Afro-Caribbean people living in Britain, but it does not seem that either group have any in-built immunity or are less exposed to factors that might cause MND. The higher life expectancy of Western populations appears to be the one consistent factor associated with higher rates of MND.

MND rates are higher in people migrating to the UK from places where MND rates are lower, and seem to be higher still in the children of people migrating here than in their parents. Ultimately they are likely to equal the higher local rate as their life expectancy also increases.

The documentary I saw recently stated that MND appears to be becoming more common. Is there a reason for this, such as more toxins being released into the air or in food?

The incidence of MND in Britain has doubled over the last thirty years, with every indication that it will continue to rise. There have been, over the years, many suggestions for possible links between the incidence of MND and environmental exposure. Suggested toxins have included industrial solvents, agricultural pesticides and organophosphate compounds. Exposure to some metals has also been implicated, including lead, mercury, selenium and zinc.

In no case have any of these tentative findings been confirmed by research. However, over these last thirty years there has been a dramatic decrease in deaths from infectious disease (some of which are now very rare or completely eliminated in Britain), and the death rate from stroke and heart disease has also declined. This has been accompanied by improvements in diet, nutrition, health care and the provision of clean water. These improvements raise overall life expectancy, and far more people now live to ages at which MND occurs (usually 50 years and older); more people therefore live long enough to be diagnosed rather than die at a younger age from other causes.

So the answer is yes, there are environmental factors playing a part in the onset of MND, but there is no evidence that the rate of exposure to toxins is the cause.

I once used a commercial insecticide in my greenhouse, and instantly felt very ill. I think this caused my MND, but my neurologist disagrees. What do you think?

If you have MND, then it is not likely that a single exposure to a commercial insecticide was the cause. MND is usually diagnosed after the onset of widespread and often unnoticed neurological changes in the body. Whilst many people with MND seem able to pinpoint an exact moment when their MND started, the onset of the disease was probably much earlier and the moment pinpointed is the first time the condition had a noticeable effect.

There is a lot of medical interest in and concern over the effects of organophosphates (OPs) on those who are exposed to them. Since they are widely used in insecticides, including most notably sheep dips, unprotected exposure to them may cause some symptoms, some of which are similar to those of MND. However, OP poisoning is not progressive unless there is repeated exposure, and the symptoms of OP poisoning do not get worse over time.

Several reports claim that MND is caused by mercury, lead and other heavy metal poisoning. Should I consider having my mercury amalgam fillings replaced with modern composites? Will it improve my symptoms?

There have been many claims about the effects of both dental mercury and of 'oral galvinism'. Galvinism is a battery-like effect of unlike metals being close together for some time (similar to the tingling sensation you experience when a piece of metal foil touches a filling). Oral galvanism occurs between different fillings with different metal contents, or between an amalgam filling and a gold crown. However, the number of mercury amalgam fillings is no higher in people with MND and it is unlikely that mercury poisoning leads to MND. There are no cases of such poisoning resulting from modern dentistry and there is no scientific evidence that the mercury in amalgam fillings is unsafe.

Amalgam removal involves the removal of all these fillings from your teeth to reduce the possibility of mercury dissolving in your bloodstream. If it is not carried out carefully, amalgam removal results in sudden, increased exposure to mercury from drilled filling fragments that you might swallow. If you are having a filling replaced routinely, you may wish to have a composite instead of amalgam and most dentists in Britain now offer a choice. There is no scientific evidence that removal of amalgam will help MND, although anecdotal stories abound of seeming 'miracles', which are never confirmed by reputable clinicians.

The effects of sudden (acute) heavy metal exposure can produce neurological symptoms very similar to some of the symptoms of MND. The theory is that people with MND either have excess metal levels in their bodies anyway, or are unusually sensitive to metal exposure (these are not established scientific facts). Many of the effects of heavy metal poisoning are reversible through treatment with soluble chemicals that attach themselves (bind) strongly to the metal – this process is called 'chelation'; these chemicals are then passed out in your urine.

I have read about mercury exposure in a Japanese population who were living near a polluted lake. Was this disease anything like MND?

This exposure occurred when a chemical factory disposed of many tons of mercury waste into Minamata Bay in Japan. Neurological symptoms including loss of motor coordination, abnormal reflexes, difficulty in speaking and brain seizures affected over 3000 people who ate fish and shellfish from the bay where the food chain included an excess of mercury. This was labelled 'Minamata disease', but the clinical picture (the sites of the nervous system affected) were entirely different from MND.

Fetal Minamata disease also affected a large number of children born to women who had eaten contaminated fish. Exposure-related disease was confirmed in Minamata residents with levels of mercury in their hair of 50 parts per million or more, which is hugely above that found normally (around 1 part per million).

It is unlikely that any resident of Britain would be exposed to sufficient mercury to cause these effects except by working in a factory using mercury or if their local environment was massively contaminated.

I have MND and my mother-in-law is terribly worried about my children catching it. Are there any special precautions my wife should take, for instance with cooking and eating utensils?

MND is **not** an infectious disease and there is no evidence whatsoever that MND can be passed from one person to another by any mechanism. For instance, MND is not more frequent among close family members of someone with MND who are not related by blood (such as marital partners, adopted children or in-laws) nor is it more common amongst medical personnel who work with people with MND. There is therefore no need for separate cooking and eating utensils, towels or washing materials.

Someone with MND may be more affected by the normal symptoms of colds, 'flu or other common infections around because of difficulties with mobility and exercise, which are important in combating and recovering from routine infections.

Trauma

I believe my MND was caused by a serious fall at work, in which I broke my collarbone, and I think that trauma plays a large part in MND. Do you think this could be right?

There was, for many years, an acceptance that MND could result from 'trauma' or injury, a term having many different meanings, even within different branches of medicine. Broadly, trauma in this case means injury to the body resulting in damage to some part of the central nervous system, and not emotional stress or shock. A large survey of American ex-serviceman with MND found more had suffered head injuries compared with servicemen of the same age without MND. The proportion of people with MND was small, however, so that, although the results looked as though head injuries were more common amongst the servicemen with MND, they could only have accounted for a fraction of all the servicemen with the disease. In addition, it is impossible to know after the event whether the head injury actually resulted from MND or that it was the other way around, namely that early symptoms of poor coordination or muscle strength caused the accident.

More recent surveys (including one conducted by the same researchers) have failed to find a similar statistically high association of MND with trauma.

Genetics

Is MND a genetic disease and, if so, are other members of my family likely to get it too? Is there a genetic test for MND to see if they are likely to get it?

The simple answer is no, there is no reason to think that your blood relatives are any more likely to have MND than anyone else.

One form of MND, amyotrophic lateral sclerosis (see Chapter 1), exists both in a form that relatives get ('familial') and a random ('sporadic') form. The familial form of ALS is associated with symptoms that start early but progress slowly; it often affects several family members over many generations within a single family. 'Sporadic' ALS is by far the more common, accounting for 90% of all people with ALS. Although genetic changes may be a cause of MND in these people, it is not clear that any risk of getting MND can be inherited by other members of the family.

If neither of your natural parents, nor any other blood relative has MND, then it is highly unlikely that your form of MND can be passed on, but equally, like any other random event, there can be more than one case of MND in a family by chance alone. We estimate that about 4% of all people with MND would be expected, by chance alone, to have a relative with MND, when great-grandparents, aunts, uncles and cousins are included as well as immediate family.

General research has been gathering pace over the last decade, confirming there is some genetic involvement in MND. About 10% of cases of ALS have a 'familial' origin, usually occurring in clusters within affected families. Outside these affected families, the familial pattern (if any) is difficult to interpret. Advances in genetic analysis have led to the discovery of 'novel mutations', in other words changes to genes following conception, but not inherited from either parent. A form of one particular gene (the superoxide dismutase-1 gene) is found in about 20% of familial cases of ALS and in some people with 'sporadic' ALS. It seems likely that MND is not associated with a single genetic cause but with a range of genes that independently alter the risk of MND and are required in certain combinations before MND is likely to occur.

It is not possible, at present, to give a genetic test to ascertain the likelihood of future MND because the two major genes already known account for only a small proportion of all people with MND. Even amongst people with familial ALS, only 20% have the variant gene (superoxide dismutase-1) associated with MND, so any test results would be, at best, inconclusive. In time it is likely that comprehensive and reliable tests will be developed.

Why do some scientists think that damage to neurones causes the immune system to react so that even further damage is caused? Is MND an autoimmune disease?

Some researchers think that MND can be accelerated and worsened by a run-away immune response mounted by the nervous system against any damage to neurones, and this immune reaction could injure motor neurones even further.

Although possible, it remains largely hypothetical, even though such a mechanism of damage to neuronal cells does occur in other neurodegenerative conditions including Parkinson's disease and Alzheimer's disease.

Because this would open different ways of treatment, medical researchers are actively involved in experiments to see if MND is an autoimmune disease, but there is no immediate prospect of changes in treatment practice or new drugs related to this research.

One of the documentaries that I have seen on the TV about MND talked about an excess of 'glutamate' killing off motor neurones. I didn't really understand this – can you enlighten me?

Since it is only the motor neurones that are affected in MND and no other nerve cells, there must be something special about these cells. The most likely explanation is in their chemistry and, in particular, the chemical involved in the transmission of messages from one nerve cell to another. These are called 'neuro-transmitters' and, although there are many of them, research has focused on a particular one called glutamate, because an excess of glutamate can kill motor neurones. Normally excess glutamate in the body is removed by an enzyme called glutamate dehydrogenase. Research concentrated on the theory that, if we could encourage this enzyme to work, this would remove the extra glutamate and, if this was the cause, stop any further damage to motor neurones. An amino acid has been tested but it has been only doubtfully successful. (See Chapter 15 *Future research into cures and causes* for more details on new drugs being researched.)

3
Diagnosis and prognosis of MND

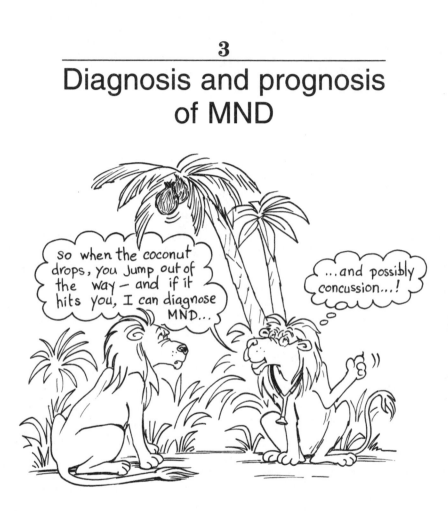

The diagnosis of MND can be difficult because there are many conditions affecting nerves and muscles, not least the effects of viral or bacterial infections producing toxins that give similar

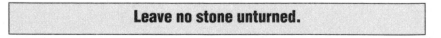

Leave no stone unturned.

symptoms. For the person with MND, the process of diagnosis can be a time of great confusion, when a lot of information has to be digested and understood. Other problems are that no single symptom alone can define MND and no two sufferers from MND have identical symptoms. Specific complaints will help diagnose MND, and some will exclude it. With repeated assessments, the diagnosis of MND becomes more certain. This may take time as the progression of motor neurone symptoms is the prime evidence supporting its diagnosis.

Diagnosis

I have been given an appointment for tests on my muscles. What will this involve?

There are five main investigations used in the diagnosis of MND, and one or more of these will be indicated:

- *Electromyogram (EMG):* This is the measurement and analysis of electrical stimuli to muscles in various parts of the body, typically the long muscles of the forearm and hand. EMG patterns show where the long and short muscle fibres occur, and where nerves might have degenerated. No needles are used (so the process is non-invasive) and is therefore painless. Tests to measure the speed of conduction of peripheral nerves ('conduction studies') may, however, be required.

- *Magnetic resonance imaging (MRI):* A series of cross-sections through the body is made using a high-frequency magnetic field that causes 'resonance', which are then reassembled as three-dimensional computer images (Figure 3.1). Because each chemical component of the body has its own resonant frequency, MRI can create detailed images of almost any non-moving tissue (such as the central nervous system) and can provide more information than CT scans.

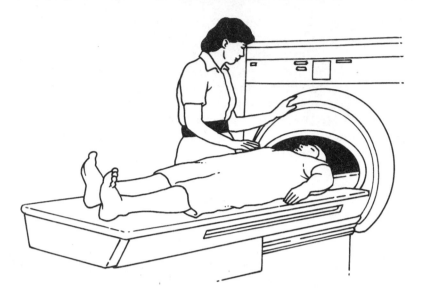

Figure 3.1 MRI scan.

- *Computerized tomography (CT or CAT scan):* X-ray images are taken through the body (mostly brain and spinal column) and reassembled as computerized data to form images that provide information not given by a single image.

- *Muscle biopsy:* This involves a minute part of a muscle being taken, using a hollow core needle, after a local anaesthetic has been given. The specimen of muscle fibres is then examined under a microscope to assess whether the fibres are degenerated.

- *Lumbar puncture (spinal tap):* A small amount of cerebrospinal fluid (CSF) is extracted after insertion of a needle under local anaesthetic between the lower lumbar vertebrae of the spinal column; the CSF is then analysed for raised protein content but normal cells that would typically indicate MND and exclude many other neurological disorders.

I first went to my GP more than a year ago, when he first mentioned the possibility of MND. Since then I have had lots of tests in hospital, but I still haven't had an official diagnosis. Why does it take so long?

MND is a condition where almost every clinical symptom is common to at least one other condition – such as multiple sclerosis, Parkins on's disease, some rare cancers of the brain and spinal cord, as well as a number of conditions causing compression or damage to the spinal cord. Since any particular pattern of symptoms may not exclude all of these other conditions, investigations do not always lead to a confident and definite diagnosis. With fewer and milder symptoms, observation may be required to see whether these symptoms worsen appreciably over time. With such a serious diagnosis as MND, no stone should be unturned to exclude other conditions and this process can take time with some uncertainty for many months.

The diagnosis will be certain only when either additional symptoms appear or existing symptoms increase in severity. This can take a great deal of time, even years in some cases, before the diagnosis is definitely MND or definitely excludes MND. It can be very helpful to record, in a diary or elsewhere, dates when any new symptom is first noticed, so that the onset of each is accurately noted for the next medical appointment.

Reactions to your diagnosis

I was not told my diagnosis. I overheard it in a conversation and then demanded to be told the truth. I feel bitter because I can't trust my doctor any more.

This situation can occur as an unfortunate consequence of the difficulty of diagnosing MND. Communicating this diagnosis to someone is emotionally distressing and doctors will naturally wait until the certainty of the diagnosis is established. This avoids upsetting unnecessarily those with suspicions of a diagnosis of

MND, which later prove unfounded. In addition, current guide-
lines on the management of MND suggest that the diagnosis
should be given by a senior doctor, in privacy, with the
opportunity for early follow-up, and that the person with MND is
accompanied by a relative or professional able to provide support.
For these reasons some time will elapse between confirming the
diagnosis and arranging a suitable consultation to communicate it.

Yours is not an uncommon complaint, and is not exclusive to
MND – for instance, some people with fatal cancers are not told
the diagnosis. This is done only when it is believed to be in their
best interests. Fortunately (except for those who do not wish to
know the diagnosis), this is becoming far less common and all
medical practitioners are as open as possible with their patients.

Doctors may guard the diagnosis from patients who would
have problems understanding it, or who might become depressed
and even attempt suicide, in the face of sudden bad news. Time is
often necessary for some to accept the inevitability of deterioration. The need for careful understanding is very important in this
communication and how it is done requires considerable thought
and assessment of the individual and their carers.

Because of this, doctors are the best equipped to provide information on the condition and the outlook for the future – so get
the most from their skills and experience.

Hope springs eternal.

**My GP doesn't seem willing to talk to me about MND in
any detail, and quite frankly I know nothing about it and
would probably be wasting his time with simplistic
questions. What can I do to find out more?**

Most family doctors will see only a few cases of MND in an entire
career and many will never encounter a case amongst their own
patients. It is natural that they cannot be immediate experts on
this condition or in a position to answer questions straightaway.
Since no one else is as well able to locate and interpret the information needed, the doctor needs time, in between visits, to think

about your questions and look for answers, and will then be very helpful. You have already made a start by reading this book yourself! You could take this book along to show your doctor.

Since the doctor's work is devoted to curing illness, they may find it hard to deal with MND, representing, as it does, such a challenge to medical skills. No question is too simplistic and so you are not wasting your doctor's time. If there is a question to ask, this means that it is important to you, and the doctor is the first person to ask about any medical matter of concern, but your doctor may also recommend someone else to talk to about your MND. Other sources of advice, information and support include the Motor Neurone Disease Association (MNDA), which covers England, Wales and Northern Ireland, the Scottish Motor Neurone Disease Association (SMNDA) and other individuals or families dealing with MND. The *Appendices* give addresses and further reading that will be found helpful.

When I was first told my diagnosis, I felt so overwhelmed that I couldn't think of any questions to ask my neurologist, but now I have so many questions that I don't know where to start. Is it possible to go back to my neurologist and ask them?

Yes. You should be able to book another consultation, through your GP, although you may have to wait a long while if you are not actually visiting for treatment – there is a shortage of specialist consultation facilities. In any case, you will probably be recalled for further tests and examinations, as well as for routine re-examination. Ask your doctor when you are likely to be seen again and request a follow-up consultation; if it is a long time before being recalled, explain how important it is to you. Private neurological assessments are readily available, but be absolutely sure of the cost of consultations and examinations before embarking on private treatment, because some neurological assessments (such as MRI scans) can be very expensive.

Since medical consultations can be short in conditions less serious than MND, it is vital to get the most from them. You should prepare questions you have in mind, preferably writing them down on paper, with plenty of space to note answers from the neurologist. Make sure that all the questions you want to ask are answered, because it is so easy for conversation to drift down other tracks. You may like to take a tape recorder to make a permanent recording of the consultation so that you can listen to it later to remind yourself of what was said or to clarify anything that you weren't sure of at the time (but do ask before recording a consultation). If you need physical help (with writing, for instance) or emotional support (for example, if you feel intimidated), then ask if you can be accompanied either by a friend, a partner or family member, but someone who is good at asking questions and staying on track. The neurologist is a professional and will be able to cope, often preferring this approach from the patient. All consultations are conducted so that a calm collected dialogue will deliver all the necessary information.

I have been diagnosed with MND, but having read a bit about it I wonder if it is possible that my neurologist has made a mistake. Is it possible that I don't have MND but have something with similar symptoms?

It can take a long while to diagnose MND – anything from a few months to a couple of years – and requires a large number of varied tests. Once a diagnosis has been established by an experienced neurologist and communicated to you and your GP, there is considerable certainty that no other condition could account for that particular range and number of symptoms.

If there is any doubt or a failure to take into account everything you know, discuss these concerns with your GP, who may be unable to answer some of the questions, but will certainly have the skills and knowledge to assess your concerns. If, after this, there are still doubts, you should ask to be referred back to a neurologist to discuss the diagnosis. In any case follow-up visits are made to assess your progress and treatment.

Essentially, if you are not getting the information or treatment you feel is needed, and asking your doctor is not satisfactory, you can and should ask to see another specialist.

Prognosis

My partner has just been diagnosed with MND. What are the usual stages of MND and how fast does it progress?

A frequent description of MND is that it is 'rapid, invariably fatal and has no cure'. Despite this, some people with MND are still alive many years after diagnosis with very slow changes in health status or levels of physical impairment. At present MND is incurable: the average survival is typically quoted as 2–5 years from diagnosis, but many people with MND live for 5 years or more from diagnosis, 10% survive at least 10 years and some rare individuals survive 20 or 30 years with the condition. (The best known example is Professor Stephen Hawking, who is reputed to have had MND for about 40 years.)

Treatments can help reduce the symptoms that lead to disability. Although there is no actual 'cure', there is now a drug riluzole (Rilutek) which is accepted to slow the progress of the disease. This acts as an antiglutamase and is given as a 50 mg capsule twice daily. Because there may be side effects, the liver enzymes are checked before and during treatment, so the medication has to be given under medical supervision. If you follow advice on exercise, physiotherapy and diet, this will also help considerably.

My neurologist couldn't or wouldn't tell me how long it would be before I became very disabled. Can you give me any idea, in general?

Your neurologist is being cautious by not stating the unknown and unknowable. There is no formula that can predict rates of progression of the disease and rates are only loosely linked to symptoms. When you have been assessed over a period of time, your neurologist might suggest that, if your MND had progressed slowly, then it will probably continue in this vein.

There is no standard progression of MND because every individual has a different course, depending on how widespread initial symptoms are and how widespread the nerve degeneration is. As a very rough rule, a wider spread of symptoms (for instance weakness on both sides, or in both lower and upper limbs), combined with bulbar palsy (for instance symptoms involving speech or swallowing), will probably cause a more rapid progression than if only one limb or the lower limbs only are affected.

I keep being recalled by the neurologist for yet another test, even though the results seem to make no difference whatsoever to my treatment. What is the point of all this effort?

Your neurologist is able to assess accurately both the degree of damage in your central nervous system and the rate of damage progress from successive tests. Tests are objective means of assessing severity, unaffected by the way you feel or the physical symptoms you experience – which are difficult to relate directly to severity of nerve damage. The point of these successive tests is to make estimates of future progression as accurately as possible in order to know how fast or slow your MND will affect you, and also where your symptoms are likely to be. This can also be an important factor in choosing the drugs that are most suitable for your type of MND.

I was diagnosed with MND last autumn, about two years after first noticing problems with walking, and so far I still have only some weakness in both legs. How long am I likely to survive?

As mentioned earlier, your own circumstances are very important in assessing an answer to this question. There is immense variation between individuals in how fast the disease progresses.

Your neurologist will be able to advise you on your own circumstances based on results of tests, the severity of your own symptoms, as well as on how fast or slow these are progressing. This is one reason for regular visits to a neurologist. Living longer is commonly associated with a diagnosis at a younger age, with a slower progression of initial symptoms, and with fewer muscles affected. This means that survival is likely to be longer in people who have slowly progressing symptoms. Survival is likely to be shorter when speech, swallowing and all limbs are affected. This broad simplification should not be taken as a foregone conclusion because individual variation is too great for such a sweeping generalization.

4
Medical treatments for MND

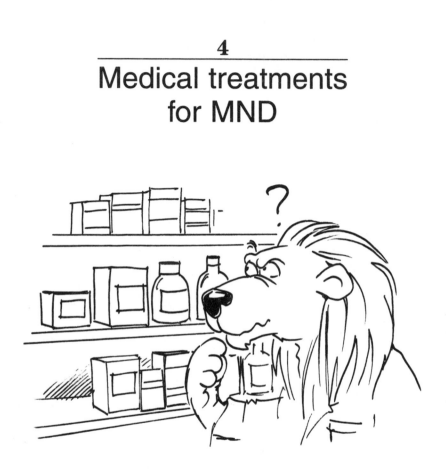

At present, there is only one drug approved for the treatment of MND itself, but other drugs are in clinical trials and may be approved in due course. Treatment therefore involves management of different symptoms to maintain your strength and abilities. The combination of treatments will vary greatly between individuals, so there is often no one correct answer to seemingly simple questions about treatment.

Drugs used in MND

My sister has been told that she has MND, but has not been prescribed anything. Are there no drugs for treating MND?

There is only one drug licensed specifically for preventing the progression of MND, riluzole (which has the trade name Rilutek). It is the only drug so far that has completed clinical trials.

Glutamate metabolism is affected in MND and it is thought that excessive concentrations of glutamate around motor neurones are toxic and result in their deterioration (see Chapter 2). Riluzole is a drug that binds together with glutamic acid, blocks its effects and reduces the concentration of glutamate around motor neurones.

Clinical trials (see Chapter 15) of riluzole showed that survival was improved in people with MND, slightly but statistically significant. In other words, riluzole does not 'cure' MND in the sense of reversing existing symptoms and restoring former health. It may slow deterioration by slowing further progression of symptoms. The effect of riluzole appears to be greatest for people with chronic progressive MND (see Chapter 1) and more limited (or not significant) in other types of MND – so riluzole is not a suitable treatment for everyone with MND. Further trials are continuing, assessing the types of MND where it might be most effective, the dosage to be given and whether the results can be improved when it is taken in combination with other drugs. In summary, riluzole is the only MND-specific treatment available, having the effect of slowing progression of symptoms in some, but not all, with MND; it is not a cure.

Riluzole is taken as a 50 mg capsule, twice daily. It should be prescribed initially by a neurologist. It should not be given to those with liver disease; liver function tests will be made before and during treatment. If the liver enzymes increase five-fold, the drug will be stopped. Other side effects include weakness,

> **Go out in good spirits with flags flying and whistle wet.**

headaches, sleepiness, abdominal upset and dizziness; these side effects are quite common with other drugs. In addition you might sense pins and needles around the mouth.

It should be pointed out that all drugs carry the risk of side effects and of interaction with other medications, should you be taking more than one. Antidepressants, for example, can be addictive and have a cumulative effect. Your body takes some time to excrete all the drug and with time you may need more and more to get the same effect as the initial dose.

My father has been told that there are no drugs to help him get better. So what is he likely to be offered then?

There are two classes of drugs or treatments that your father's doctor will discuss with him. The first is the wide range of effective treatments for individual symptoms, not necessarily confined to MND. Drugs for difficulties with excess saliva for example are discussed in Chapter 7 on *Problems with swallowing and breathing*. Others are mentioned in the appropriate sections.

Some drugs, not developed specifically for the treatment of MND, may be effective for some aspects of MND because of their 'side effects'; for example, antidepressants such as amitryptiline have the side effect of drying up saliva in the mouth, which can be useful for the treatment for excess saliva in MND.

Other sorts of treatment aimed also at slowing or halting the progression of MND include antioxidants and creatine.

- **Antioxidants** are widely available in a number of forms and are easily obtained from any chemist or health food shop. They include the vitamins C, E and beta carotene (widely available in combination as a once-a-day vitamin supplement for stressful lives), in health supplements such as green tea, grape seeds and garlic, as well as in food items such as oily fish, fresh fruit and fresh green vegetables.

- **Creatine** is a food supplement that can aid the growth of muscle mass and stamina after exercise. Designed to be used in athletic training programmes, it is claimed to have a beneficial effect in slowing the progression of MND. It is also available widely in health food shops.

None of these approaches has been confirmed by clinical trials. Both of these supplements are discussed in Chapter 6 on *Complementary therapy and self-help in MND*. There is considerable research for future drug treatments and these are discussed in Chapter 15 *Future research into cures and causes*.

Other treatment choices

My doctor has offered me physiotherapy sessions. Should I take these up?

Physiotherapy is important in helping to reduce the physical disabilities caused by the progression of MND. Your physio-therapist will assess your mobility and devise a schedule for you

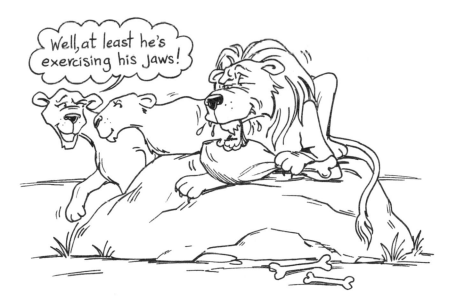

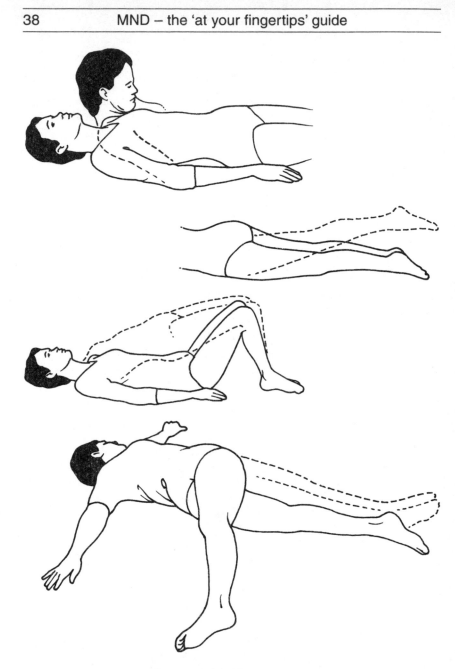

Figure 4.1 (a) Floor exercises.

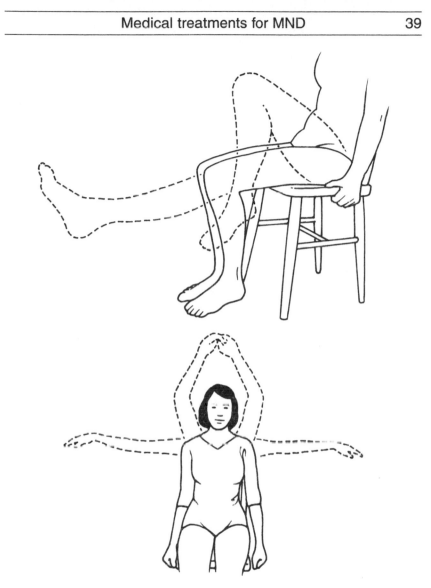

Figure 4.1 (b) Chair exercises.

that will most probably include a combination of active exercise (Figure 4.1a, b and c) and passive therapy, where someone else, initially your physiotherapist, helps you to move beyond your previous capabilities (Figure 4.2). The physiotherapist will also

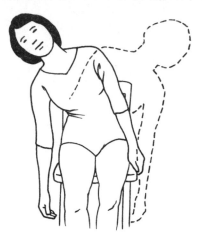

Figure 4.1 (c) Chair exercises (continued).

advise on safe and unsafe activities (e.g. the safest way to lift heavy objects, enter the bath or turn when washing), provide some training for members of your family and other helpers, and tell you about the wide range of aids that can help with your mobility. The physiotherapist may be the first person to talk to you about walking aids and wheelchairs, but occupational therapists (see below) can also help here. Physiotherapists have

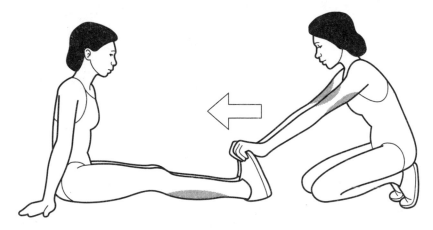

Figure 4.2 Passive stretching.

a great deal of experience helping with mobility problems – the goal will be to reduce the impact of debilitating symptoms.

I often experience difficulty in making myself understood now. Could I get help?

Yes. A *speech therapist*, despite the title, is involved not only in all aspects of speech, but also in helping you to swallow and breathe. A speech therapist is particularly important in bulbar-onset MND (see Chapter 1) where speech and swallowing are affected early, and can advise on the best ways of dealing with swallowing liquid and solid foods. There is more about help for speech in Chapter 8 *Problems with communication* .

I have had sessions with a very good physiotherapist and she has told me that I would benefit as well from occupational therapy. What is the difference between them?

An *occupational therapist* is concerned with activities of daily living such as dressing, eating and bathing. When fit and healthy, we often do things in quite clumsy ways without even noticing because they are well within our capabilities, and an occupational therapist is skilled at spotting this 'habit' behaviour. Your occupational therapist will want to observe how you perform specific tasks to assess your coordination and skills, in order to suggest other easier ways of doing them. Advice will be also be offered on aids and adaptations that will help you in the home, work or elsewhere. These include adaptations to bathrooms, dressing and washing aids and devices for cooking and eating. These are all discussed in Chapter 10 on *Adapting to life with MND*.

I have become very depressed recently and my doctor has suggested I see a counsellor. Will she be able to help?

Counsellors can help you, as well as your family, with the many emotional and mental problems that have to be faced with MND – from coping with the diagnosis, to adapting to life with MND, and the changes in family relationships that are likely to occur. Many of the ordinary and everyday stresses that are trivial without MND can become much more serious as the condition deteriorates. Whoever acts as your counsellor – be it a priest, social worker, therapist or doctor – they can make a great deal of difference to your ability to cope. We discuss this further in Chapter 14 on *Coping with MND*.

5

Surgery for MND

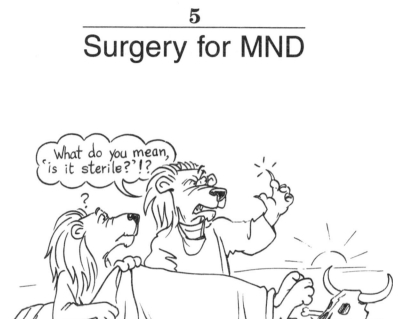

The are two operations performed in people with MND: 'tracheo-stomy' and 'gastrostomy'. Some surgical interventions have been used in the past, e.g. laminectomy for spinal decompression, which are now known to have no value in MND. Some people with MND benefit from successful foot surgery to correct foot alignment. Although bladder problems are rare in MND, some people may require a suprapubic catheter fitted, which does not interfere with sexual intercourse. All surgery in MND is aimed at alleviating disabilities only, not at curing the disease itself.

I have breathing problems and have learnt from my GP about surgery to help with this. What is she talking about?

The operation for breathing problems involves a *tracheostomy* – an opening (stoma) is made from the front of the throat into the windpipe (trachea). The incision is made under local anaesthetic and a tube can then be inserted to help breathing, usually with the aid of a 'volume ventilator'. A suction tube may also occasionally be inserted through the same opening to remove mucus and other secretions. This is usually done at the same time as the breathing tube is removed for regular cleaning. (We discuss breathing problems further in Chapter 7.)

My wife has reached the stage of needing to be fed automatically. Can you tell me what the surgery that her doctor has offered her is all about?

Surgeons will make a *gastrostomy* – an opening made in order to pass a feeding tube straight into her stomach. The technical term for this is a 'percutaneous endoscopic gastrostomy' and it is sometimes called a 'peg' for short. The feeding tube is left in place all the time, for as long as 6 months, between cleaning and replacement. Food will be administered by a pump either continuously (drip-feeding) or as intermittent meals (bolus feeding). Your wife might be offered this instead of 'nasogastric tube' feeding, where a thin plastic tube would be threaded through her nose and down into her stomach for feeding.

I have noticed that one of my feet is not 'working' properly any more. Is there anything that I can have done to help me – I am loathe to use a wheelchair if I can help it.

Before you get to the surgery stage, you could try bracing or a corrective device. Mild foot drop or foot deformities can be corrected with braces. Braces will maintain proper alignment between your foot and leg. This will improve your mobility and walking ability while reducing the risk of sprains and other injuries. (If you have similar problems with your wrists, you could use splints for support and alignment.)

If your foot drop is more severe making it impossible for you to walk without dragging your foot, this can be corrected with an 'ankle–foot orthosis' (AFO). This surrounds your ankle to hold your foot in correct alignment. Both braces and orthoses prevent muscle contractures (permanent fibrotic contractions) and their resultant deformities. Contractures can form in the knees, hips and ankles. They particularly affect the tendons at the back of the ankle (heel cords, Achilles tendon).

Persistent foot deformities that develop may need surgery. This can release persistent tension in your tendons, which prevents joints from returning to a relaxed position. Fusing two or more bones together can also help improve stability (arthrodesis).

My husband will be going into hospital soon because he has such problems with urine incontinence. What will happen to him?

He may already have had an intermittent or indwelling catheter. An indwelling *suprapubic catheter* is inserted surgically through the wall of his abdomen (tummy). This operation is suggested for medical reasons (because of other conditions that may be preventing entry through his urethra, or because of infection) or because it is more convenient. Life could become significantly easier, particularly with regard to not needing any help to empty his bladder, self-cleaning or regular re-insertion that accompanies intermittent catheterization. He will feel a lot better about himself and it shouldn't interfere with your sex life together. There are risks of leakage of urine around the catheter opening and the suprapubic catheter will need to be removed again after some months or years. Both types of catheter (intermittent and indwelling suprapubic) can cause infection in the urethra and bladder.

When I went to my doctor for information on surgery, he told me that I would have to pay privately for it. Can't I get these operations done on the NHS?

Although you probably feel that surgery might help your problems and would significantly increase your quality of life, some operations listed here (particularly foot surgery and suprapubic catheterization) could be regarded as 'elective' procedures in the UK, operations that you choose to undergo rather than operations your doctor thinks are necessary. As a result, this sort of surgery is not widely available and may not be available under the NHS. If you think that you would benefit, your doctor will be able to refer you for an opinion from a private surgeon but, as a private patient, you would have to pay both for consultations and treatment.

6
Complementary therapy and self-help for MND

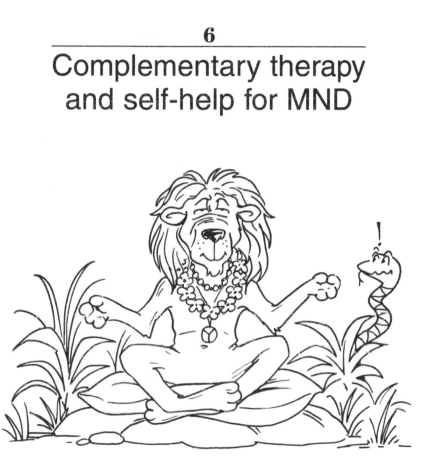

There are a wide variety of practitioners of complementary, alternative, traditional and natural therapies working outside the mainstream healthcare system. The qualifications and credentials of these practitioners range from higher degree level and membership of an appropriate association, to no qualification whatsoever. There are few laws governing such practitioners and anyone can describe themselves as a therapist and offer treatment to the public. Having said that, there are established registers and qualifications for almost every complementary therapy, and therapists should willingly tell you their qualifications and membership of relevant societies.

Few complementary treatments have been proven safe or effective in clinical trials and are therefore generally regarded as 'unproven'. On the other hand, few clinical trials have been undertaken at all, largely because there is no incentive to test any therapy that cannot later be patented and marketed for profit. There has been a notable increase in referrals from the mainstream healthcare service to complementary therapists since the rise of budget-holding GPs, so clearly some doctors are at least satisfied that complementary medicine can reduce drug bills and therefore costs. Whilst these referrals may be simple cost-saving, it is also true that many medical treatments are almost completely ineffective (such as, for example, the treatment for long-term back pain) and alternative therapies are at least as good. An alternative explanation for the increase is that, as there is no cure, any treatment gives hope and is better than no treatment at all.

Keep the patient involved, informed and updated.

People keep telling me all the right things that I should be doing to maintain my health, but what about all the things I should avoid? Should I refuse inoculations, try to avoid ordinary infections (like 'flu) and medicines like antibiotics?

Largely, you should do the same things as everyone else – inoculations (such as the 'flu vaccination) are more likely to prevent a bout of 'flu than cause an adverse reaction, so there is no real reason to avoid this sort of inoculation. A bout of 'flu (or even a severe common cold) is likely to affect those with MND far more than it would affect someone who does not have the condition, so it is sensible to avoid catching colds and 'flu. Most winter infections are transferred by bodily fluids, so try to avoid kissing (even a peck on the cheek), make sure that people don't cough or sneeze around you and don't share glasses or cups – all these precautions reduce your exposure to infections.

Antibiotics, on the other hand are designed to eliminate existing infections; if you have been prescribed them, the consequences of not taking them could be serious illness or worse. Serious risks occur, particularly in ear, abdominal and urinary tract infections. Unfortunately, antibiotics have been prescribed for trivial conditions such as minor throat infections, and conditions that do not respond to such drugs, such as viral infections like the common cold. Since they may cause unpleasant side effects such as nausea and diarrhoea (caused by the elimination of your own 'useful' bowel bacteria), antibiotics should be avoided if possible. If your GP tends to overprescribe antibiotics, don't be afraid to ask whether the side effects might be worse than waiting to see if the infection runs its natural course.

Vitamins and supplements

My doctor mentioned the importance of a balanced diet and how some vitamin and mineral supplements can help achieve this, but which are the right ones to take?

Most people living in Western Europe have a diet containing adequate quantities of all essential nutrients and minerals. It is essential that your diet is balanced and contains plenty of fresh ingredients, especially fresh fruit and vegetables, and does not contain excessive fats, especially solid fats. Some people claim to benefit from additional 'antioxidant' vitamins C (which is unlikely to have any adverse effects), E and beta carotene. If you benefit from vitamin C supplements, then you would benefit even more from increasing your intake of fresh fruit (especially citrus fruits like oranges), sweet peppers, tomatoes and brightly coloured vegetables, such as peas, beans, Brussels sprouts, broccoli or parsley. These food items also contain dietary fibre, an essential component of healthy digestion and bowel function.

Do not take any of the vitamins in excess, especially vitamin A. Vitamins A, D, E and K are fat-soluble substances that can be stored in the body (and some are released very slowly), and produce overdosing. Vitamin A should be avoided during pregnancy as it can produce birth defects. These vitamins are not rapidly excreted in urine (as are the water-soluble vitamins, such as vitamin C) and can therefore accumulate to excessive and harmful levels when vitamin supplements are combined with an adequate dietary intake of vitamins A and D. Serious side effects can also occur from too much intake of minerals in your diet, such as iron.

My muscles have weakened considerably. Are there any body-building supplements to help preserve the strength and tone of my muscles?

Body-building and athletes' food supplements are designed to promote muscle mass in combination with strenuous exercise, in other words to accelerate or intensify the effect of a rigorous training schedule. There is no evidence that body-building supplements will have beneficial effects in the absence of exercise. The human body is well able to excrete, through the bladder and bowel, any nutrients that are not used within the body. Indeed, any dietary excess of such supplements can put a strain on liver and kidney function. There is also evidence that some body-building supplements are manufactured to poor standards and can have harmful effects.

One supplement that has received a lot of attention recently is creatine, a component in the manufacture of muscle fibre within the body and now a 'functional food' used by athletes and body builders in training. There are claims that it can slow the progression of MND, and there is anecdotal evidence for this; there seems to be little evidence of harmful effects of this supplement when obtained from quality suppliers. Creatine is undergoing clinical trials as a therapy for MND, after which the value of claims will become clearer – the compound is, of course, already widely available as a food supplement in health food shops.

Diet

I have heard a lot of talk about diet having a positive influence on MND. Where can I find out more about the right diet to follow?

The right diet to follow is a healthy, well-balanced diet, and there is no evidence that any special 'MND diet' will improve symptoms or slow its progression. Most people's regular diet could always contain more natural fibre, fresh fruit and vegetables, and antioxidants (vitamins C and E particularly). Others may benefit from a reduction in red meat and alcohol consumption.

Information about diet is available from a wide variety of sources including your own medical advisers, organizations for people with MND, and the internet (a number of websites are listed at the back of this book), but always remember that the right diet is a sensible diet. There is no control over the content of documents on the internet – so it is possible to find both useless and harmful advice in web documents. Finally, you can ask your GP for a referral to a dietician.

Complementary therapy

The range of therapies available is too wide to cover in a book such as this, although we have tried to give a broad overview. In general, the range of therapies is broader and therapists are easier to find in big towns and cities than in rural areas. There are few forms of therapy that are not available somewhere in Britain.

There are several therapies that people with MND have claimed to be helpful or useful, although the value is often in coping with related problems (such as not being able to relax, or stress) as much as in helping the symptoms of MND. Nobody has ever been cured of their MND by any of the therapies discussed below, although some people have claimed to be significantly helped.

How can I choose a competent complementary medicine practitioner?

All practitioners, whether mainstream or complementary, should be qualified by an acknowledged organization of some form. They should normally offer evidence of their training if asked, and may have certificates on display or have accredited letters after their name. Many of the accrediting organizations are listed at the back of this book. In some disciplines (chiropractic, for example) the usual level of qualification may be a university degree or postgraduate diploma. The appropriate national organization will be able to tell you the minimum standard that they expect of a practitioner offering treatment to the public, and will be able to tell you if any individual practitioner is registered with them.

There is usually more than one body representing some practices, all claiming to be the principal national organization, but any one practitioner is likely to be registered with only one of them. These bodies will vary in the rigour with which they enforce qualification and practice standards. Be aware also that there is no legal requirement that complementary practitioners are qualified to practice or qualified to use the title (e.g. doctor or consultant) that they use.

There are a growing number of holistic and alternative health centres acting as a focal point for practitioners and often providing clinic space for a variety of different therapies. Whilst these centres cannot be relied upon to provide independent recommendations (they are, naturally, more likely to refer to their own practitioners than to practitioners elsewhere), they are a useful contact point and source of information. Wholefood shops and health shops also tend to know of local practitioners and often make available complementary health newspapers that advertise therapy.

Acupuncture

This is a treatment involving minute punctures of the skin by thin needles to stimulate nerve endings underneath the skin along lines of *Qi*, or energy flow, according to ancient Chinese principles. The needles are left in or stimulated for up to 20 minutes. Acupuncture has been used by people with cancer for pain relief and instead of anaesthetic during dental procedures. It has also been found to alter blood supply and change the release of chemical transmitters in the body to alter mood and muscle stiffness.

I have decided, after talking to friends who have benefited, to try a course of acupuncture. How do I go about finding a good, reputable acupuncturist?

If you know other people who have used and would recommend an acupuncturist, then this is certainly one of the best ways to find a practitioner. Unlike many other therapies outside the medical mainstream, acupuncture has gained considerable respect in Britain, which means that your own medical advisors may well know of practitioners in your area.

You can also find acupuncturists through the British Medical Acupuncture Society – the address and contact details are given in *Appendix 2*. You can also check that any individual acupuncture practitioner is qualified with the British Medical Acupuncture Society.

It is sometimes possible to receive acupuncture directly through the NHS.

Aromatherapy

My wife often has an aromatherapy session to help her relax after the stress of looking after me. Do you think it could help me too?

Aromatherapy (which you can also practise yourself) is a treatment intended to invigorate or relax you to aid recovery and healing. We don't think anyone can dispute the positive effects of a pleasant soak in the bath or a massage with a soothing aroma of essential oils, extracted from flowers, herbs, spices, and woods, but practitioners claim much deeper effects.

Oils are diluted with a carrier oil (such as grapeseed, almond, avocado or sunflower oil), at about 5 drops per 10 ml carrier oil. Positive effects are claimed, for example basil or bergamot for depression; lavender, neroli, camomile or sandalwood for stress, or ylang ylang for anger. It is important to use essential oils rather than the cheaper scented oils used for pot pourri or oil vaporizers. Never apply these essential oils directly to your skin in an undiluted form because they can cause skin irritation. Advice can be obtained from a pharmacy, health food shop or any good book on the subject.

Osteopathy

I am about to have a series of osteopathy treatments. Is it very different to chiropractic?

Osteopathy regards the musculoskeletal system as a unified whole, critical in maintaining health. Thus bones, muscles, connective tissue and nerves all play a part in the symptoms of disease and in fighting disease. Disruption of any part of the system can have consequences elsewhere – we have all heard, for instance, how a badly fitting pair of shoes can lead to back pain or headaches in addition to sore feet.

Osteopaths use various forms of manipulation, stretching and the application of pressure to restore movement to joints, attempting to rebalance opposing muscle groups in order to alleviate pain and discomfort. Qualified osteopaths are registered with the General Council and Register of Osteopaths.

Chiropractic, on the other hand, is directed almost exclusively on spinal column alignment and flexibility in the vertebrae (discs).

Chiropractic

Chiropractic treats spinal posture and is possibly the most cost-effective treatment for some back pains and related problems (although this is still hotly contested amongst mainstream doctors). Chiropractic involves the manipulation (as in bending and twisting) of vertebrae and joints to increase their flexibility. Be absolutely sure that your chiropractor knows that you have MND and to expect your muscles to be weak, in order to avoid any injury.

I have been using a chiropractor since before I was diagnosed with MND and have found that the treatment helps with my mobility, but it is expensive. Is there any way that the NHS would pay for it?

At present the NHS will not provide chiropractic centrally as a preferred treatment for any condition, including MND. There is a slim possibility that your local GP practice, which is able (within certain constraints) to spend their budget as it chooses, might provide chiropractic if doctors believe it to be at least as effective as, and cheaper than, other treatment that you are having under their budget. In other words, a GP practice can use chiropractic (or indeed any other therapy) to save money, so long as the quality of care is maintained.

Homeopathy

The administration of a minute dose of a compound that, in larger doses, gives the same symptoms as the condition being treated is called homeopathy. The reaction to the compound is intended to stimulate and amplify your immune system and healing responses of the body. Some people allergic to bee stings, for example, have minute injections of bee venom over a period in time, which eventually can lead to an immunity against a bee sting. Another example is where a toxic compound (that would normally cause a fever when taken in high dose) might be diluted many, many times to a harmless dose to bring down a temperature.

There's a local homeopathic centre near me, which I hear has very good results with all sorts of conditions. Could homeopathy help me?

It is unlikely that any homeopathic therapy would have an effect in slowing or reversing the progression of your MND, but many people do claim that it is effective in treating many conditions that are both common and distressing in MND, including 'flu, colds, stomach upsets and muscle cramps. Since no other treatment has been claimed to be an effective cure of the common cold, it could indicate that homeopathy is at least as good as anything else in your local pharmacy! Since few people report side effects with homeopathic remedies, if the treatment does help some of these conditions, then mainstream drugs that might have uncomfortable side effects have been avoided.

Yoga

Yoga exercises have a deep spiritual meaning for people who follow the discipline seriously. Exercises involving mental self-discipline ('clearing the mind'), breathing exercises and relaxation, combined with an emphasis on posture, could be useful to many people including those with MND. Yoga helps many people with breathing and swallowing difficulties – but in MND speech therapy should take priority.

Somebody at the local branch said yoga was very helpful for their MND, but I wonder how it would actually help?

Yoga is taught at various levels, from simple relaxation techniques involving no faith, to a deeply spiritual practice that becomes a way of life. While yoga is not normally part of a religious belief system (although individual practitioners may be, for instance, Hindu or Buddhist), it is not usually perceived to conflict with religious belief (Christianity or Islam, for example).

Meditating can be much easier that you might think. Teachers will show you how to concentrate on your breathing, which will take your mind off 'mind clutter' and lead you to a feeling of deep calm. The yoga exercises involve the mental discipline to clear all conscious thought, making the mind more receptive, breathing more controlled and posture good. Meditation helps relaxation (and therefore coping with stress), breathing and swallowing. As a result, whatever level yoga is taken, it may help some with MND.

Hypnotherapy

Hypnotherapy is today a much more recognized form of healing, using a combination of counselling, mind analysis and hypnotic techniques. A skilled therapist helps to alleviate many problems of a physical or psychological nature by inducing a state of deep relaxation which is claimed to allow direct communication with a person's subconscious mind.

Reflexology

Reflexology works on the hands or feet, 'unblocking' blocked energy pathways. The therapist's sensitive hands can release tension and improve circulation. Reflexology tries to heal the 'whole' person, not just symptoms of the disease.

Other alternative treatments

You hear about such weird and wonderful complementary treatments. Some seem really way out, but do they help?

Apart from the more accepted forms of complementary treatments mentioned above, there are indeed a few that some might call 'weird'. These include:

- *Magnet therapy.* This has been claimed to cure almost everything, including migraine and rheumatoid arthritis, but there is no scientific evidence of any healing effect, and certainly not in MND.

- *Venom treatment.* This has appeared at various times as a

treatment for MND and occasionally has been used with
pseudoscientific justification of its value. The two most
popular toxins have been snake venom and bee (or wasp)
venom. Some of the toxins used in venom therapy have
contained chemicals related to compounds in clinical trials,
but natural compounds tend to be taken in uncontrolled
doses and are adulterated with compounds with completely
unknown effects.

We do not think that treatments like these should be tried until
more scientific proof is available that they can help.

7

Problems with swallowing and breathing

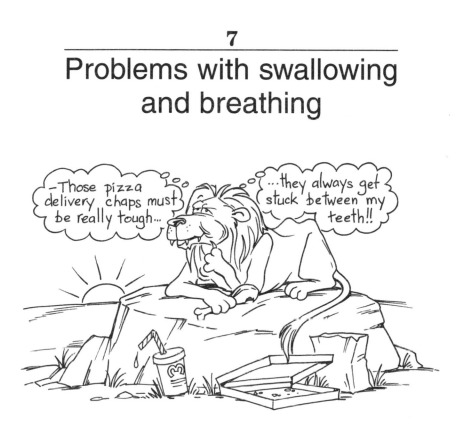

Since breathing and swallowing impact on every other activity and every relationship in some way, problems with them are two areas of MND that can be potentially distressful, causing discomfort, embarrassment and humiliation.

Health professionals are familiar with these problems and can help considerably, so ask all the questions that are needed, no matter how trivial or ludicrous they might appear, and be open about your fears. Benefit will be most obvious after sorting out these everyday needs as early and as thoroughly as possible.

Swallowing

The team that can help with swallowing difficulties includes a dietician, speech therapist, physiotherapist and doctors at various times depending on the associated problems with eating, drinking, staying active, communication and mobility.

I am producing a lot more saliva in my mouth than I used to and, apart from the embarrassment of dribbling, I am afraid of choking. Should I drink less fluid or something to reduce my saliva?

It is not excess production of saliva that causes the problem, but rather the difficulty of swallowing the saliva, which leads to excess saliva left in the mouth, and then dribbling. Saliva is a healthy component of the digestive system, containing enzymes that aid bowel regularity and the breakdown of food. The first approach in controlling excess saliva is to maintain a good posture and adequate breathing. The speech therapist will be able to advise on both, as well as on other matters that can hinder swallowing, such as the type of food to be eaten.

The intake of fluids should **not** be reduced, as good fluid intake is necessary for adequate bowel function and good health. Reducing fluid intake does not, in any case, affect saliva production.

Are there any drugs to help with this problem of dribbling?

If excessive salivation is still a problem, then excess saliva can be reduced by drugs.

The production of saliva can be reduced by anticholinergic drugs such as hyoscine, atropine or glycopyrrolate (normally prescribed for drying secretions prior to general anaesthesia, for irritable bowel syndrome, Parkinson's disease, slow heart beat, asthma or urinary incontinence); tricyclic antidepressants such as amitryptiline (normally given for depression, anxiety or insomnia); or a beta-blocker (usually given for high blood pressure, angina, irregular heart beat or for protection against further damage after heart attacks); all these drugs are available on prescription only and have the useful side effect of drying the mouth. In all cases, there will probably be a period of dose adjustment in order to select the lowest dose that has an adequate effect, or choose an alternative treatment.

A portable suction device (like those machines that a dentist might use) can also be useful for removing excess saliva.

What can I do about the choking mucus that builds up in my throat?

Preparations like Robitussin may help reduce thick phlegm and clear the airways generally. As with any medication, it should be used according to the patient leaflet or under the guidance of your medical advisors, who may suggest other medications, such as Vick or steam inhalers (which are really best for nasal rather than lung congestion) especially if you need to use them for a prolonged time or frequently.

More importantly, your normal sitting, eating and sleeping positions will need to be assessed to minimize congestion and maximize your ability to breathe and swallow. The best source of guidance and advice on these issues is a speech therapist or dietician.

Eating used to be such a pleasure, but the difficulties my husband has now in eating without help make it impossible for him to enjoy his food and mealtimes any more. He always used to be so independent and it is hard for him to ask for help all the time. How can I remove the frustration for him?

First, it is important to set aside sufficient time for eating, without distractions such as other family members talking (or arguing!) and the television. If eating in silence is not comfortable, then talking books, radio plays and music are suitable entertainment that would not affect his concentration too much

– and are a good way of establishing a regime for eating. As well as getting the ambience right, it is important that your husband has the right place to sit comfortably and reach everything that he needs when he wants it. This might also mean, for example, providing an extra gravy boat or serving dish of vegetables, so that it can be left within reach rather than asking someone to pass it to him. Give him plenty of space too so that he will be able to pick up and put things down without dropping them, or knocking other crockery or glasses.

It is better to have more frequent, shorter meals – there is nothing worse than having one main meal a day, which your husband is always going to be eating cold because he doesn't eat as fast as everyone else. Taking hot soups and starters well before a meal, and hot puddings some time afterwards, can help because he will be able to eat a manageably smaller dish.

Difficulties with eating create an opportunity to experiment with foods that are both convenient and enjoyable. Your husband could try eating fish and chips, thick-slice pizza or chicken thighs with his fingers, for instance, or stir-fried foods (which are, necessarily, pre-cut before serving), casseroles, curries and other saucy foods with manageable chunks in them. Mashed potato, polenta, Arborio rice (which is much stickier than long grain rice), couscous, bulgar wheat and short pasta will be easier for him to eat than roast potatoes and long spaghetti. The traditional meat and vegetable or Sunday roast are, unfortunately, probably the least convenient of all dishes.

I have a lot of trouble now in enjoying soup, which I have always loved, as it is so difficult to transfer the spoon to my mouth without spilling any. Do you have any suggestions?

Apart from using special crockery and cutlery (see Chapter 10 *Adapting to life with MND*), it is always possible to thicken a finished soup using cornflour – a teaspoonful of cornflour made into a paste with a tablespoonful of water and stirred into simmering soup should be more than enough to thicken one portion of soup. Plain flour can also be used, but it has a tendency to form lumps and will alter the flavour more; it can be added (usually to butter or oil) at the start of making homemade soups. Cooked pulses, such as lentils, or cooked vegetables, such as potato, can also be used to thicken a soup, and can be blended first. If added uncooked to the ingredients of a homemade soup, they will need at least 30 minutes cooking time. Most supermarkets also sell thickening granules containing a fat (either suet or vegetable fat) and cornstarch, and these can be added directly to any simmering sauce, gravy or soup without the risk of lumps because it is preblended. This might suit you if you prefer your soup or sauce thicker than the rest of the family.

I have never liked swallowing pills, even as a child. Now that I have to take them to preserve my health, is there any way of making them easier to swallow without choking on them?

One method that many people use is to place a single pill on the back of the tongue, near to the throat, and then drink a swig of water or milk, which should wash the pill down without even being noticed. Alcohol does not mix well with drugs, and might reduce their effects. Fizzy drinks can make swallowing even more difficult.

You can put your pills into a spoonful of jam, honey or béchamel sauce if preferred, because none of these will lessen their effects in the least. Ideally, whatever you put them in should be fairly thick and palatable, and something that you enjoy eating for its own sake.

If necessary, you can grind up hard pills and remove the contents of gelatin capsules so that they blend with other food. Sometimes the contents of a gelatin capsule are either bitter or foul tasting and are far less agreeable than the gelatin capsule itself. That is, after all, why the drug company chose to use a gelatin capsule to put them in!

If you do blend a pill with other food or drink and do not consume it, you must be sure that it is thrown away to avoid the risk that someone else might consume the medication by accident.

Breathing

I am terrified of choking to death – I wake up at night frightened that I won't be able to breathe, and then stay awake.

Although this is an everyday fear for many people with MND, the reality is that there is very little risk of choking to death (asphyxiating). An episode of choking and its associated fear can be very disconcerting. It is good to raise these fears with your doctor, speech therapist or dietitian, to see what practical steps can be taken. For instance, Robitussin has sometimes been recommended for loosening excess and thick phlegm in order to ease breathing, although not all people agree it has a useful effect.

I frequently feel very short of breath. Is there anything that can be done to help me take deeper breaths?

Shortness of breath may come on after exertion such as walking or talking, although it can occur without obvious reason. Relaxation and rest will restore deeper breathing naturally, but breathing exercises can help improve and maintain good breathing. Taking pressure off the diaphragm also allows deeper breaths:

- Sit in a chair with your feet firmly on the ground, about a shoulder's width apart and lower your chest towards your knees. Allow your arms to fall straight down if it is comfortable and does not strain your back unduly; otherwise rest your elbows on your thighs.

- Sit on a chair at a table (dining table height is about right – the height of your elbows when sitting bolt upright) and lay your head on the table using a cushion or other article for comfort.

Once you have found a comfortable position that permits easy deep breathing, you can exercise your lungs to maintain capacity:

- Inhale as much air as you can, so that your lungs are comfortably full.

- Hold the breath for anything from a few moments to a half a minute, as you feel able.

- Exhale as fully as you can (once you think you have finished exhaling, exhale some more).

- Repeat from 2 to 10 times.

Documentaries from Japan and the USA about MND showed many people using mechanical ventilators. I haven't been offered this help here. Why not?

Mechanical ventilation is more frequently used in some countries than others, although documentaries exaggerate the differences because people featured in documentaries about MND are often unusual or exceptional in some way. Using an invasive mechanical ventilator is a major step for someone with MND and is often seen as a permanent sign of disease progression. It will take over your breathing and manage your diaphragm and delivery of air to your lungs. There are three other devices that might help:

- Non-invasive positive pressure ventilation (NIPPV) is now more commonly used in the UK.

- Oxygen, in a cylinder with an attached mask and a regulator, can provide a great deal of relief by enriching the air you breathe and making shallower breathing more effective at getting oxygen into the lungs. Oxygen can be helpful in eliminating tiredness and headaches even if you have only slight problems.

- A Bi-Pap is a dual-pressure device that helps you to breathe, particularly during rest and sleep, by maintaining a pressure difference, allowing airflow into the lungs with less effort from the diaphragm muscles.

I often wake up feeling tired and short of breath. Is there something I could do to help this?

This may be a result of you shallow-breathing (hypoventilation) during the night while lying down, which requires more effort than breathing while sitting or standing. As muscles, including those of the diaphragm (which control breathing), become weaker with MND, they will tire more easily and perform less effectively. This can be overcome to some extent with simple supports and changing the relative height of your diaphragm. You could use additional pillows, a wedge-shaped support under your head and shoulders or even raise the head end of the bed. If the bed is not designed to be raised, then the legs at the head end can be raised with wooden blocks, by about a hand's width.

I get very depressed with my choking and breathing problems every day. Are there any drugs that might help me?

Sometimes a combination of the drugs diazepam, diamorphine, chlorpromazine and hyoscine prescribed by a doctor might ease your symptoms. Full information on breathing difficulties and treatment is available in the form of the *Breathing Space Kit*, available from the MNDA (for address see Appendix 2). The kit needs to be completed with drugs prescribed by your own doctor and should be kept for emergency use only (see the question on tracheostomy in Chapter 5).

8

Problems with communication

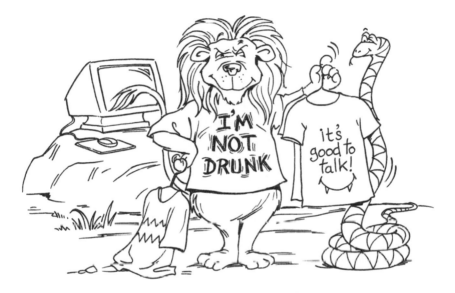

Problems with communication for people with MND are very diverse. They include the direct effects of the condition associated with muscle control, weakness and shortness of breath. Less directly are the difficulties associated with other activities, such as eating, where talking during a meal may interfere with swallowing. Not least is the changing family and social patterns imposed by the need to speak slowly, being bed-bound or in a wheelchair – even the difference in the physical height of a wheelchair can be a barrier to comfortable conversation. Technological developments, especially the home computer, have added to the wide range of aids, and there are many purpose-made machines such as the Possum range of communication and control devices, the portable Canon Communicator or the Lightwriter. For social obstacles to communication, the essential answer is to allow time and space and adapt activities with family and friends to enable communication at a slower pace.

> **Understand a suffering shared is a suffering halved.**

Interaction with friends and relatives

Since my speech was affected, my family don't take the time or trouble to involve me in conversation anymore, which is terribly isolating. How can I get more involved or command attention, as I still feel I have as much to offer as I ever did – maybe more since I have more time to think about things than I used to!

Adopt an equal position. Most importantly, you need to be in a position that doesn't relegate you to the background – if you are seated in a chair or lying in a bed away from conversation, then you will not be participating equally, no matter how hard everyone tries. The solution could be as simple as moving the television, if that is where everyone sits, to bring you into the arena, or turning the dining table so that you are not sitting behind people. Sometimes it can be much more difficult, and will involve altering the entire way in which your family uses the spaces in your home – perhaps in terms of eating or sitting elsewhere.

Avoid distractions and interruptions. Television itself often dominates the family environment. Most of the time, we cope with TV, everyday activities and conversation with apparent ease, but when we are tired or ill, it suddenly becomes a strain to cope with interruptions and distractions. This is especially true in order to overcome an initial inertia in getting ready to talk, and the need to maintain momentum once you start speaking. In this situation, even small distractions can put a stop to your participation in conversation. Try to eliminate these by, for instance, switching off the television for a part of every evening (especially mealtimes, when there is a tendency to meet and chat as a family), or even placing the TV in another room.

Try planning more for conversation. If there are news items in the paper or parts of books that you want to share, have them ready so that it doesn't interrupt conversation while you look for them. Make sure the conditions are favourable and the right people are present for conversation. If you want a quiet, adult chat, then starting when noisy children are present is not a good idea. Similarly, if you are having a serious conversation that requires concentration, don't start it minutes before the washing machine goes into its spin cycle.

Use visual cues more. If it takes you a while to formulate a sentence and get started saying it, develop some sort of gesture that indicates to everyone else that you are about to speak – it could be as simple as raising a hand or finger. Of course, everyone else has to learn to wait and listen in response, so it may take a while to work effectively.

Particularly where children are involved, it may be useful to obtain impartial and independent advice on problems that hinder effective communication within the family. Family counselling provides a mutually safe environment in which members can examine the family situation and their individual roles. Counselling encourages family members to explore problems openly, to express feelings and to adjust flexibly to changing roles. Counselling can help develop a better understanding of effective listening and establish boundaries in relationships and behaviour. See more about counselling in Chapter 14 *Coping with MND*.

I have developed palsy and get really mad when sometimes people think that I am drunk when they hear the way I speak. Is there a polite way of putting them straight?

Short of wearing a T-shirt saying 'I am not drunk – I always talk like this', there isn't a polite response to people who judge you on sight or sound, without thinking about it. If you are interested, a lot of shops can make up T-shirts with printed messages to your order, or you can buy iron-on T-shirt transfers that you can print with a computer printer at home.

If you don't mind carrying a message card, then you could carry a postcard in your pocket saying that it is difficult to speak or that your speech is difficult to understand, but that you are going to speak anyway. If you show the card before you speak, then nobody in their right mind would think that you are drunk, and you shouldn't be concerned about offending people who don't wish to understand.

Simple aids

Paper and pencil

I would like to find something cheap, small and dependable for my wife to help her communicate with others when we are out. She treasures her independence, so it has to work with strangers too.

If your wife can still write, then the simplest, cheapest, most dependable and lightest of all communication devices is a pencil and pad of paper. The most useable pads are probably spiral-bound shorthand notepads, with lined sheets bound at the top and a stiff cardboard cover on the back. A soft pencil of B or 2B grade writes well in all conditions, including rain (unlike a ball-point) – but remember to give her or take with you a sharpener or spare pencil. A mechanical propelling pencil, the ones with loose leads pushed out by a button, never need sharpening. A few sheets of paper with useful messages used frequently can save a great deal of writing and paper, and can be made very durable with a self-adhesive clear plastic coating.

If writing is difficult because hand control is not good, but still possible, then a larger pad of paper will prove useful. If your wife is right handed, then restricting her writing to the left of the page will help, leaving a hand-width right margin to support her hand (and conversely, a wide left margin to support a left hand).

Combine this with either felt-tip pens or crayons that can support some hand and arm weight without piercing the paper.

My wife is still as bright as a button after many months bed-ridden with MND and always loves doing crosswords and puzzles, but she finds it hard to manage them now with her weak arms and hands – especially as magazines seem to be getting thicker all the time. She would be so happy if someone could find an easy way of doing them.

Magazines are indeed becoming weightier and more full of advertising than ever before. If you don't intend to keep the magazines, then cut them up to separate the pages of interest. For crosswords or puzzles, use a tray as a firm surface to hold both the magazine cutting and a pen or pencil – trays with bean-filled cushions that stay level on a lap or other uneven surfaces are ideal. You can stop the magazine cutting from slipping by fixing it to a sheet of firm cardboard cut to fit the tray. A glue stick or an aerosol can of artists' spray mount are both neat ways of sticking cuttings down. The sticky top edge from Post-It notes is a re-usable method of sticking, as is general-purpose masking tape. Artists' mounting board is a good surface to stick paper to for writing on, but it tends to be a bit expensive.

A soft (B or 2B) pencil or a fibre-tipped pen is easier to write with than ballpoint pens. As well as having the advantage of not getting gummed up the way that ballpoints do, they can support more weight without damaging the paper.

If the crossword is too small for your wife to cope with, then it is always possible to make enlarged photocopies on plain paper. This can make it easier for your wife to fill in the boxes, as well as being much easier to see at a distance.

You can adjust the lightness of the text and the contrast between dark and light on many photocopiers. Black and white photocopying of A4 sheets (about the size of an ordinary magazine) costs a few pence and is widely available in corner shops, newsagents and libraries. Colour photocopying costs more, but is unlikely to be necessary unless the magazine has printed text and background of different colours that are equally dark. If you have a home computer with a scanner and a printer, then you should be able to make your own copies easily and cheaply at home.

Speaking typewriter

My mother has MND and has been unable to speak for a long while now. At home we are all set up with a speaking typewriter, and she can even call for help (and interrupt other people!) with the volume turned right up. Are there any new models of this type?

These devices are usually called communication aids or, more specifically, electronic speech aids. Technology is evolving very fast, and now there are also software communication packages for portable Windows CE computers and for various Personal Digital Assistants (PDAs) like the Palm Pilot. As a result, anything we write here will probably already be out of date by the time you read it. You can get reliable, up-to-date information about newer communication aids from your speech therapist or local speech therapy department, from AbilityNet or from the various communication aids centres across the United Kingdom, contact details for which are in Appendix 2.

There are several names (for instance Possum, Cambridge Adaptive Communication, Toby Churchill [Lightwriter], Prentke Romich and Sunrise Medical [Dynavox]), which have all produced speech aids and continue to bring out new products. The capabilities and prices of these products will act as a benchmark to judge anything new, or to judge PDA-based software products. The MNDA and SMNDA run a useful equipment loan service. Contact details are also given in Appendix 2.

Features to look out for are whether the device runs from batteries, and how long the battery lasts between charges when fully used (i.e. with the display switched on, and speaking at a moderate volume continuously, rather than in standby mode); whether a car adapter (or wheelchair battery adapter) can be used; how easily the vocabulary and settings can be customized to an individual (e.g. with names of friends and of favourite foods or activities); how loud the maximum volume is without distortion; and how light and useable the device is in practice (e.g. can your mother switch it on, or set the volume and other settings without help).

Morse code

A long-lost army officer friend visited us recently, and I was amazed to find that my father (who was a telegraph engineer) could tap out Morse code, which his friend could understand and reply to. None of us knows any Morse code and, short of learning it, is it possible to 'translate' it into text through a computer?

There certainly are pieces of software that can interpret Morse code and turn it into text on the screen. One such is Morse Code WSKE (Words+Software Keyboard Emulator), but there are others, including some public domain and shareware software for Morse code training and amateur radio enthusiasts. The best place to look, if you have a computer and internet access, is on some of the search engines for "Morse code". An occupational therapist may also be able to suggest alternatives, because Morse code is not the most efficient keyboard replacement available, although knowing it already must be a big help.

A Morse code reference card, which you could write yourself on a postcard, and a notepad to write the text would probably be even better. You will probably be surprised how soon you can pick up enough Morse to be able to understand basic questions and answers. The notepad with both Morse code messages and their corresponding text would act as a useful reminder of frequently used words. You would probably be able to dispense with the notepad very quickly and simply reply with a best guess of the message. Morse code has the advantage that it can be used anywhere you can tap or hum, which a computer does not have.

Speech aids

I should like to know what technical devices there are to help with my speech, which is getting poorer – there seems to a bewildering selection!

On the technical front, the number of devices available can seem bewildering and there are constant changes as newer, lighter speech aids come on to the market. Electronic communication aids that are light and portable have three basic forms of output – speech, text on a screen, or display and text on a paper tape. The two critical factors for your purpose are likely to be the weight and the battery life between charges – bear in mind that speech aids are usually designed to rest on a wheelchair, not to drop in a pocket.

You should be able to get the latest information about speech aids from your speech therapist, from such organizations that deal with disability technology as RADAR (the Royal Association for Disability and Rehabilitation), from patient support groups like the MNDA or SMNDA, or from the manufacturers themselves. See Appendix 2 for some addresses.

Note that there are sometimes exhibitions of communication aids at meetings such as the MNDA or SMNDA annual general meetings, which are usually held in a single-level or disabled-friendly venues with good hotel and transport facilities, such as the National Exhibition Centre (NEC) in Birmingham.

Telephone-type aids

Using the telephone is something I find increasingly frustrating, because it tires my arm and shoulder so much, although I am finding the phone more and more important in my life. Are there any modern telephone aids that might help?

There are plenty of different devices: some you can use with your existing telephone, some are easier to use, and there are also completely different means of communication that work through your telephone line. Since deregulation of the telephone system and the abolition of the telephone monopoly, there are many more companies making and selling telephone equipment and services. The traditional telephone shop is still around, and an excellent place to look at telephone equipment and pricing, but telephone equipment is also available in department stores and catalogue shops.

If you have a fairly standard telephone, especially the one supplied when the telephone line was fitted, then you can definitely benefit from a change of phone. Telephones are available with big, readable push buttons that make dialling easier, and with memory functions to store frequently used or emergency numbers – these can be written on labels on the phone. Handsets now come in a wide range of shapes and can be much lighter than standard phones – a lightweight, large handset is probably the easiest to handle. Handsets with the buttons built into them (all-in-one phones) are probably the most difficult to manage. Some people like to use a self-adhesive shoulder rest for the handset, which lets you tuck the phone between cheek and shoulder without the need for using hands at all.

The ultimate in easy telephone use must be a loudspeaker phone, such as seen in an office setting. Although more expensive than a standard telephone, it allows dialling and two-way conversation through a built-in microphone and loudspeaker that can be used within about 3 metres (10 feet) of the telephone, without the need for pressing any buttons once you have dialled out or picked it up.

Lastly, a wireless telephone can be carried around without any wires and has the keypad built in (although they are often small) so that calls can be answered or dialled from anywhere in the house. The latest digital equipment cordless telephones (DECT) have a much greater range (about 60 metres [200 feet]) and less noise from interference. These telephones are like mobile phones but linked to a base station plugged into your phone line. New features include call transfer between up to five handsets on one line, paging, intercom, text messaging, simultaneous internal and external calls and conference calling.

My daughter wants me to get a mobile phone, but I am not sure that the expense (especially the call charges) could be justified. What do you think?

Even the simplest mobile phones have facilities far exceeding what can be done with a home telephone. Imagine, for instance, having a phone with a headset (microphone and earpiece) that you can use to dial someone simply by speaking their name, a display that shows you who is calling before you answer, that accepts both recorded and written messages from your friends while you are busy, that you can wear discreetly wherever you go, that plays recorded music or the radio when not making a call, and lasts all day on one battery charge. This is all possible now, although it might have absolutely no appeal for many people. The advantages of a mobile phone include:

- Mobile phones work anywhere and fit in a pocket, take only an hour to recharge, give a few hours of calls (or a week on standby) from a single charge – and you can always be contacted at the same phone number, wherever you go, sometimes even on holiday abroad!

- They contain an address book with names and phone numbers that simplify calling frequently used numbers and record those rarely used numbers that might be needed when you are away from home. Some mobile phones also have facilities for storing notes and diary appointments.

- The Short Message Service (SMS) text is a method of sending a text message to another mobile phone, like an electronic mail message. Messages are received immediately by the other person if their phone is switched on, and they will be received later on if the other person is making a call or has switched off their phone. This means that people can read and respond to messages when they feel like it and don't need to interrupt what they are doing to answer the phone. Many people with mobile phones use them only for sending and receiving text.

- Mobile phones increasingly use predictive text input. On most phones, the letters of the alphabet are typed by pressing the number keys several times, cycling through 'ABC' on the '2' button for instance. Predictive text speeds up input by guessing which word is being typed, although mobile phone keys can be very small and difficult to manage. The alternative is a phone with an alphabetic keyboard, or a keyboard add-on that is available with some models of phone.

- Hands-free kits consist of a headphone and microphone, so that you don't have to hold the phone. If the phone also has voice dialling, then you can start a phone call by speaking a preprogrammed phrase (e.g. a friend's name) that the phone will recognize.

- Some mobile telephones can be adapted with a plug-in keyboard to simplify writing text messages. Mobile phone contracts can permit free or reduced rate calls between subscribers within the same network or telephone company.

The two disadvantages of mobile phones are their size and cost. The cost has to be balanced against the advantages and, for some people, mobile phones have no advantage or are too fiddly to operate. There is no mobile phone suitable for use by people with poor finger control, because the buttons are too small, too close together and too stiff. There is also no mobile phone suitable for use by people with even moderate visual deficiencies because the displays are too small and lack contrast. The first manufacturer to make a large mobile phone with easy-to-press buttons and a clear display will obviously be on to a winner.

The salesperson in the telephone shop mentioned a Minicom. Is this worth trying?

If you have difficulty being understood on the phone, then you can send written messages to another telephone number. You can send typed text from one Minicom phone to another Minicom phone using the built-in keyboard and display, but you do need two of these appliances to send any message at all. Of course, mobile telephones can also be used to send SMS (short message service) text messages (see previous question) or email between specialized telephones (WAP – Wireless Applications Protocol). WAP empowers mobile telephone users with wireless devices to access easily and interact with information and services instantly. These telephones basically are the very modern ones with a built-in web browser.

Would it be worth me buying a fax machine?

If you have a fax machine (and the prices are now much lower), then you can send typed text, letters or news clippings to other people with a fax machine. You can fax any black and white image that could be photocopied, including scribbled writing and sketches. Of course, you can only fax messages to people with fax machine themselves!

Computers

My husband can no longer manage his beloved typewriter and would like to find a less exhausting method of writing letters and keeping in touch with people. I wonder if a computer would help, but I don't know anything about them and I am confused by the sales people in the shops. My husband is also discovering that he is something of a poet, so it would mean so much to him to find the right system!

Computer keyboards are certainly lighter on the hands than manual typewriters, and computers have the benefit that work can be saved, changed and reprinted as many times as you like. This means that you can save a lot of typing by re-using standard parts of letters that you have written before. You can also use different typefaces and put pictures into the text.

Before buying a computer for the first time, find someone whom you know and trust and who has one at home to demonstrate to you. Be sure to watch them explain the whole process from switching it on, starting up some software (a word processor is the software used for typing text), through to saving the document and printing it out. This will give a good idea as to the sort of questions to ask in the shops. If you have a computer-literate friend to take with you to the shop, all the better as they will be able to interpret the strange language that computer salespeople speak.

Don't go overboard on the first computer you buy – they are all much the same in use – and don't let yourself be forced into buying all the added extras on offer. If you want a computer specifically for typing (word processing), then even the cheapest and most standard Windows or Macintosh computer with a printer will do what you want and much more.

You might consider buying one of the new voice-activated computers. These are more expensive so do find someone 'in the know' before you buy one.

You will need to plan where you are going to put a computer at home. Have a look at other people's computers in their homes or at work to see just how much space they take up. They are never as small and neat once at home as they were when set up in the shops. Once all the power cables, printer cables, loudspeakers and so on are connected up, they occupy a space the size of a kitchen table, about 1×1.3 metres (3×4 feet) of desk space at least.

Laptops

As a suggestion, a laptop or notebook computer has very few cables, has the screen and keyboard in one small unit and can be taken from room to room with little trouble. Despite the name, they are not comfortable on your lap and not as portable as they look once you include the power supply and other accessories. Whatever the salesperson says, they only work for a few hours from batteries and really need to be plugged into the mains for useful work. A good quality laptop can be used with a full size, extra keyboard, a mouse and a standard display (just like a desktop computer) for ease of use (as the laptop keyboards tend to be smaller than normal), but you will have to pay for these separately. Laptops are more expensive than standard machines.

Video phones

The video phone of science fiction is now a reality, so if you want to see or be seen by someone else with the same device then you can buy a pair – they are at present sold only in pairs. Do not expect television picture quality from a telephone line. The images are black and white and do not refresh as rapidly as television images, so pictures are a bit jerky.

Internet

The internet is another way of using a telephone line. A computer with a modem and an account with an Internet Service Provider (ISP), often your phone company or computer supplier, would allow you to send email, fax messages, voice messages, pictures and video, according to what equipment and software your computer has installed. There are even software programs that perform video phone calls or 'whiteboard' calls where people scribble or write messages on each other's screens. It is important to see any of these applications in use (preferably in the home of a friend or acquaintance) in order to see what they can do in real life and how easy or difficult they are to use. Above all, look at how much space is used by computer equipment, as it is sizeable.

9

Problems with bladder and bowel function

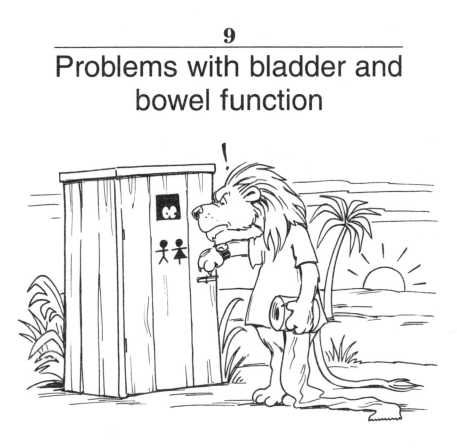

Whilst bladder and bowel control are not affected directly by MND, changes in mobility and eating patterns can lead to problems with constipation and difficulty in using the toilet when needed. In addition, help from other people when using the toilet, or even discussing problems related to using the toilet, can be a source of embarrassment. Always remember that medical professionals have seen and heard it all before and are there to help, and that getting toilet problems sorted early will save a lot of effort and difficulty in the long term.

Bladder

Is there a simple, safe way to help me use the toilet when I choose and avoid needing to go when I don't want to? I am worried about diuretics and antidiuretics interfering with my other medications.

The safest way of regulating the time needed to use the toilet is by regulating the quantity and timing of what you eat and drink. Everyone should have an intake of at least 2 litres of fluid per day, but the time at which this volume of fluid is consumed makes very little difference. It is probably most sensible to drink liquids at about the same time as eating (but don't alternate mouthfuls of food and sips of drink because this makes digestion more difficult) and immediately after waking, when most people are slightly dehydrated. Other than that, make sure to leave plenty of time between drinking and planned activities that could be spoilt by needing the toilet too often. This includes not having a large drink immediately before bed if night-time trips to the lavatory are a problem.

Bladder training involves a schedule of using the toilet at particular, convenient times so that your body becomes used to the ritual, and (most importantly) sticking to the same times every day even when you don't feel you need it. Your physiotherapist will be able to advise you on whether pelvic floor exercises (such as those expectant mothers learn in antenatal classes) would also help. The pelvic floor muscles support the bladder, urethra and rectum. It is easy to find these muscles by tensing them to stop the flow of urine while urinating. Once you know where they are and how to tense them, you can exercise this area by contracting, holding for a count of 6 and then relaxing them. Do 20 contractions up to 3 times a day – the exercise regime (called Kegels) is effective for women and men, and can be done while walking, standing or sitting during normal daily activities.

Note that some drugs used to treat symptoms of MND (particularly anticholinergic drugs and tricyclic antidepressants) will modify the urge to use the toilet and have an impact on its timing. In general, drugs are rarely the best way to deal with continence problems, but it is possible that the side effects of other therapies could be beneficial for you (for instance by regularizing your schedule of bladder voiding). You should discuss possible side effects of any drugs currently taken, along with possible variations in the times they are taken.

I find I have great difficulty getting up in the night to go to the toilet, and often wet the bed. I am deeply embarrassed by it. Is there anything that would help?

Some foods and drinks have a diuretic effect (i.e. they make you urinate more frequently), especially coffee, cola, chocolate and alcohol, resulting in an increased frequency or volume of urine. Some foods and drinks act as bladder irritants and increase the urge to urinate; these include fizzy drinks, dairy produce, tea, coffee and other caffeine-containing drinks, citrus fruit juices, tomatoes, spicy foods, artificial sweeteners, sugar and sugary foods. These should all be avoided last thing at night before bed. Regularity is very important in bladder management. In the case of night-time urgency, this would mean always using the toilet before bed, at the same time every day, even on those days that you don't feel the need.

Constipation can lead to bladder incontinence by increasing the pressure on the bladder, so that it feels unbearably full. Dealing with bowel problems (usually with a strict bowel regimen and suitable dietary modification) can sort out this type of bladder incontinence as well.

Incontinence pads are a very useful way of protecting clothing and bedding from minor accidents. Light pads have a waterproof plastic backing with adhesive strips that stick to underwear and can be worn in clothing day or night. A heavier insert pad can be used for more serious wetting, but is worn in a pouch inside waterproof pants. Both forms of continence pad are very discreet and can be worn under even very lightweight clothing without any visible sign, so they are as useable during the daytime as they are at night. A waterproof undersheet can be used to keep the mattress dry and protect it from stains.

Finally, there are NHS Continence Advisors who have access to various shapes of urinals, which can be used in bed or in wheel-chairs. Do ask your GP to refer you to one or contact one of the suppliers such as Incontact or the Continence Foundation (see Appendix 2 for details).

Every time I pass urine, it hurts. Is this yet another symptom of MND? Is it serious?

This is not a symptom of MND and might even have nothing to do with your MND. It sounds like it could be a urinary tract

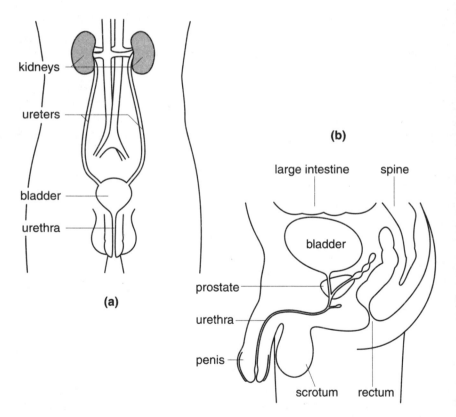

Figure 9.1 Urinary system (**a**) and lower urinary tract (**b**) in the male.

infection, a simple, easily treated infection of the urethra and possibly the bladder (Figure 9.1), characterized by a pain ranging from mild discomfort to a severe burning sensation. Urinary tract infections are very common, especially amongst women and amongst people with reduced mobility. Treatment with antibiotics is simple and effective, so you must see your doctor to discuss your symptoms. Drinking more fluids helps to relieve the pain on urination and reduces the likelihood of further infection. Increasing the acidity of the urine also inhibits bacteria and can be achieved very simply by drinking cranberry juice or vitamin C supplements.

Left untreated, a urinary tract infection can progress to an infection of the ureters (the pipe-like tubes linking the bladder to the kidneys) or kidney infections, which can be serious infections when associated with reduced mobility. A kidney infection (pyelonephritis) is often accompanied by pain in one or both sides of your lower back (loins), and this pain may spread to your side or groin. There may also be muscle aches and pains or shaking chills. These more serious conditions may initially result in apparently mild symptoms including lethargy, mild fever and a general feeling of being run down that can last for weeks or months before the cause is recognized and treated.

Bowel

Toilets are my biggest problem, because I dare not go any-where unless I am sure that I will be able to find useable facilities. I know it's a funny question, but are there any guides to public toilets?

There appears to be no single, comprehensive guide to all toilets open to the public, but lists and guides are available from the organizations that provide public toilet facilities. These include local councils and corporations who run public toilets, as well as such private organizations as shopping centres, chain stores or chain restaurants that provide toilet facilities for their customers.

Private provision has improved considerably over the years, although still very variable, and there are several reliably good chains that have a similarly high standard of toilet provision in all their branches. RADAR (the Royal Association for Disability and Rehabilitation) offers a key service to provide excellent toilets for the disabled or wheelchair users in all kinds of locations.

There are also details of facilities in most guidebooks to hotels, restaurants, pubs and inns, visitor centres, tourist guide-books and National Trust houses. These will usually state whether facilities are disability/wheelchair-accessible, as well as whether wheelchairs are available on loan and whether paths are level. See Appendix 2 for some addresses.

I always find that I am unable to empty my bowels when I want to go to the toilet, but end up uncomfortable and in need of the toilet when it is impractical or impossible to find one. How can I control my bowel more – I used to be regular, every morning.

MND does not affect how your bowel works or your anal sphinc-ter, which controls bowel movements, but lack of mobility has a large effect because exercise helps your bowel to work properly. Sometimes the pelvic floor muscles can be affected, which makes it difficult to pass faeces. Changes in diet, the amount of chewing when you are eating, and saliva production are all important parts of digestion. Ideally all food should be reason-ably firm and chewed many times, absorbing enzymes from our saliva during chewing, as these are an important element of the digestion process. Mashing, puréeing and processing food all reduce the degree of chewing and the amount of saliva produced, which reduces the efficiency of digestion and can cause constipa-tion. Constipation and bowel irregularity are actually very common in our modern society owing to the increasingly poor diet that most of use indulge in, and we would all benefit from:

- a diet high in natural fibre (bran, most unprocessed cereals, fruit and vegetables), which assists the formation of a good volume of easily transported stools;

- well-washed raw vegetables, which are better than boiled vegetables and digested more slowly (steaming or microwaving vegetables until just tender is a better alternative to boiling as this preserves most of the structure, vitamins and natural goodness of raw vegetables);

- plenty of fluid, especially water, meaning at least 2 litres (at least 6–8 glasses) per day (but do not drink in between mouthfuls of food as this reduces saliva production and reduces the efficiency of digestion);

- a reduction in the intake of bowel irritants including coffee, alcohol, highly spiced foods and sugary drinks or sweets.

There are some bulking agents (e.g. Fibogel, Metamucil and Mucasil) available, which are easily used supplements to assist with regular bowel motions (fibre pills in gelatin may suit some people). Stay as mobile as possible and ensure regular, daily movement of some kind, combined with making time for regular bowel habits.

10
Adapting to life with MND

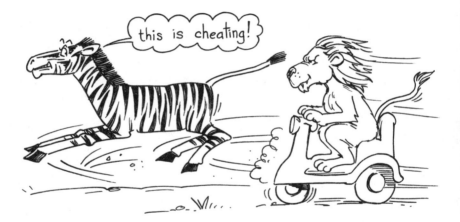

Although MND is a variable condition, affecting each person in a unique and distinct way, it is very consistent in the manner that it affects a broad range of everyday activities In this chapter we discuss some of the activities of daily living (ADLs) that are affected by MND and solutions to some of the most frequent difficulties encountered. The areas discussed include issues of mobility, dressing, bathing and feeding.

Mobility

My husband is not nearly as mobile as he used to be, although we do get him up and help him with exercise every day. He is now very sore, especially on his buttocks and thighs, which are very red. I understand that these are bed sores, but wonder what we can do to help?

These do indeed sound like the beginnings of bed sores, or pressure sores to give them a more accurate description. Pressure sores arise from restricted blood flow with consequent lack of oxygen and nutrient supply to the affected skin and underlying tissue. Because of long periods of sitting or lying in bed or in a chair, the blood vessels to the skin are compressed with infrequent relief of the affected area (Figure 10.1).

Pressure sores are not inevitable, and a range of devices, dressings and strategies exist to relieve continuous pressure. Your doctor or health visitor will be able to advise you on relieving pressure and preventing pressure sores using techniques including:

- changing position (from sitting to lying, from lying to sitting, or from one side to the other) frequently and certainly at least every 2 hours; ensure that you have physical assistance if you need it because turning or moving your husband could put a huge strain on your own back and risk serious or even permanent injury – your physiotherapist will be able to advise on the most practical techniques;

- making use of proper pressure relief devices, including support cushions and seating, to maximize the area of skin in contact with the support and thereby minimizing the pressure;

- rolling or lifting instead of sliding when changing his position, to prevent friction damage to skin and underlying blood vessels;

- keeping the skin area clean and dry, especially if urinary incontinence or leakage is a problem – the ammonia

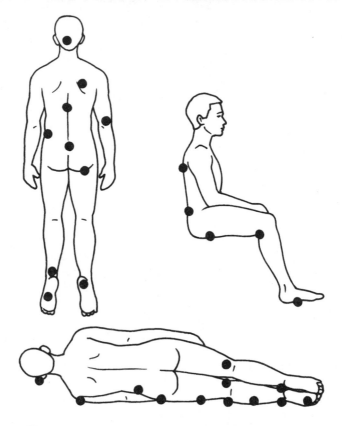

Figure 10.1 Areas where pressure sores can develop.

produced by urine causes serious irritation of the surrounding skin;

- making sure he drinks an adequate amount of fluid and has a good diet to preserve a healthy skin condition.

I have MND and I am mobile and reasonably fit, considering. Is it safe for me to continue regular exercise?

Absolutely. So long as the exercises are sensible and safe, there should be no problem. Light to moderate exercise including walking and swimming are ideal, and exercises that get you breathing well will maintain your 'vital capacity', the size and strength of the lungs. Exercise will not make your symptoms worse, although you will find it tires you more than it used to, and strenuous exercise is not advised. You are bound to find that it will take longer to recover from exercise but, if fatigue is affecting other activities, then you are probably overdoing it.

Exercise in moderation will really help to preserve both muscle mass and muscle tone in the long term. Take the time to discuss both exercise and physical therapy with your physiotherapist. It is also important that your physiotherapist instructs someone else (a family member, a friend or your carer) in how to help you with your exercises for the times when your therapist is not available.

If your muscles are significantly wasted (atrophied), then range-of-motion exercises are important to maintain flexibility, whether these are 'active' exercises that you perform yourself or 'passive' exercises that need a helper to assist you with the actions. Significant, tiring exercise is not recommended for atrophied muscles. (See Chapter 4 for an illustration of some exercises.)

I should like very much to get out of the house more with my wife who has MND – she enjoys being out and seeing new things, but it is so difficult with her wheelchair. Are there any decent guides to places that are wheelchair friendly, like historic houses and gardens?

It is always difficult to know in advance what 'wheelchair friendly' means to different people, so you may find that some privately owned places of interest claim to be wheelchair friendly but, in practice, are nothing of the sort. Fortunately for people in Britain, many historic places of interest are owned by just three organizations.

- The Royal Horticultural Society (RHS) owns and maintains a wide range of gardens open to the public, and organizes special events for members.

- The National Trust and English Heritage between them own and maintain a large number of historic homes and estates across the country, most of which have good accessibility – particularly to the gardens and grounds, but less so within the buildings themselves.

It is often impossible to modify historic homes with listed status to provide access to upper floors, so you will still find that not every part of every site will be wheelchair friendly. All three organizations publish excellent guides detailing just how wheelchair accessible their sites are – guides and addresses are given in Appendix 1 and 2. The ratings tend to be very consistent, so you will have a good idea of what to expect when you arrive.

Some sites, particularly those with large formal gardens, offer wheelchair and power scooter loan and this can save a great deal of effort in getting ready to go – it is always wise to telephone first to check availability.

Wheelchairs

We have a wheelchair that was supplied through our local authority, which my husband uses quite a bit, but it is heavy and fairly uncomfortable. The worst problem for me (I am not very tall or very strong) is getting the thing into the back of the car. You don't exactly see wheelchairs in the shops, so where could I go to find something easier to handle?

You should be able to get good advice about wheelchairs from your occupational therapist or physiotherapist, to whom you can be referred by your GP if you have not been referred already. There are also a number of Mobility Assessment Centres or Wheelchair Service Centres operating within some Regions of the NHS. The occupational therapists and other team members in these Centres carry out detailed assessments of mobility needs and are well acquainted with all the available equipment, including that not normally available within the NHS.

The manufacturers of wheelchairs can also provide detailed information about their own products and provide comparisons with other products. The range and usability of wheelchairs has improved dramatically in recent years, due in no small part to the interest in and support for sports activities for people with disability. Independent advice, as for any sizeable purchase decision, is essential.

You may be eligible for help with part or all of the cost towards a 'standard' wheelchair within the mobility portion of the Disability Living Allowance (DLA). You are not likely to be able to top up any financial award to which you are eligible in order to pay for a more expensive chair of your own choice. You can get general information leaflets about the DLA from your local Post Office and specific further information about eligibility in your own circumstances from the Benefits Agency. Additional advice is available from DIAL, the Disability and Information Advice Line, and MND support organizations listed in Appendix 2. Note also that the MNDA and SMNDA may offer loan services in some circumstances.

Can you make any general recommendations about self-powered wheelchairs or electric cars?

Many people who have powered chairs believe that they could not get by without them, and they certainly are wonderfully liberating in the degree of independence that they can bring. In general terms, the following points might be useful for choosing a powered chair:

- Once you have chosen an electric car or chair, don't expect to combine it easily with other forms of transport as you can with a folding chair – electric chairs are too heavy to lift, do not fold, do not fit in a standard family car and can be almost impossible to get onto train platforms or buses – so you may need a standard chair as well. However, it is possible to buy powered lifts or lightweight ramps to enable you to raise an electric wheelchair into the back of a hatchback or estate car; if you intend to do this, make sure that the wheelchair services are aware, because some adjustments may be needed to the chair. It is worth looking at the whole package of car/wheelchair/lifting device together, and plan for the worst possible scenario! Some newer larger taxis will take the smaller powered chairs.

- The battery life, in terms of the average distance it would be possible to travel on full charge, will vary greatly between chairs, dependent on the weight of the chair or car and the size of the batteries. Typically you should expect a few miles travel from an overnight (8-hour) charge.

- A powered car with a full lighting set is permitted on a highway (road) and therefore does not suffer the inconvenience of having to get up and down kerbs. Even so, electric cars do not require a driving licence.

- Whilst you can travel a fair distance in an electric car, some can be isolating because of the low level at which the driver sits. If you wish to talk to passers-by or walking companions, then you may find some of the high level electric scooters more suitable.

- Some people might find that a bicycle (or tandem with a peddling partner in the lead or behind supplying some push) or a tricycle is even better than an electric chair. Modern adult tricycles are excellent for shopping trips and for longer distance travel.

Dressing aids

Is there any way I can help my husband button his shirts more easily, without hours of fiddling for him?

There are a few solutions. A buttonhook is an old-fashioned device that looks and works a bit like a crochet hook – you push it through the buttonhole from the front, wrap it around the button and pull the button through to the front. Be sure that the handle is thick enough for your husband to grip comfortably. If his shirts are big enough (and loose fitting is fashionable now), then see how many buttons he can do up before he puts the shirt on. It should be possible to do up both cuffs and all except the top three or four front buttons. If he lays the done-up shirt on a fairly high, flat surface, he can slip both arms into the sleeves and then raise both his arms to put it on like a vest or pullover. Yes, we all know this is lazy and crumples the shirt – but there are far better ways to spend time than doing things the proper way, especially when nobody else is going to see!

Another simple solution is to avoid buttons on new clothes as much as possible, even to the extent of removing them from his existing clothing. You could enlarge the buttonholes and sew on larger buttons if there is sufficient fabric, or you could sew the buttons on the front of the shirt (over the buttonholes) and sew a strip of hook-and-loop or a zip inside. This isn't possible with formal shirts because of the collar button, but works well enough with casual wear. Velcro, zips and pop-studs (especially the big ones) are all easier to handle than small buttons. Loose-fitting track suits, cotton pullovers and jump-suits are all fashionable and involve no buttons at all. Better still, they don't involve any ironing either!

Despite my legs and arms being much thinner than they were before I developed MND, I seem to have developed a paunchy belly which grows during the day. If I wear trousers which fit properly in the morning, then they feel uncomfortably tight by the evening but, if I wear comfortable ones, they tend to fall down.

A lot of us feel the effect of slackening muscles as we tire or relax, and the apparent growth in our midriffs that can be very uncomfortable in some clothes. Trousers with elasticated waists are the best as they grow with you, but stay snug enough not to fall down – track suits and jump suits are good, especially those with a draw string that can be adjusted. A spring toggle on the drawstring is easier to handle than tying a bow. Alternatively, wear trousers a little loose and use an adjustable belt to keep them up, or, even better, wear braces, which will not require any tightening around your waist at all.

Is there a good alternative to shoe laces, which I find so difficult to do up now because I don't have the reach to tie them or the strength to tie them tight enough to stay done up?

Slip-on shoes and shoes with Velcro fasteners are very popular, as are sandals with snap-locks or buckles, so it should be possible to find new shoes to suit you. Slip-ons should stay on with no fastener, so getting shoes in the right size is more important than with fastening-type shoes. There is more choice in sports and casual shoes than in formal footwear, and sports shoes do offer excellent grip, support and comfort. Golfing shoes tend to be more expensive than sports shoes, but they do have a classier look about them than runners or trainers. A shoehorn is a great help in putting shoes on, but get one with a long handle so that you can put shoes on while you are seated in a chair, and avoid bending down.

There are helical elastic laces that can be put into laced shoes instead of ordinary laces – the theory is that you pull the two ends out straight, against each other, to open all the coils, and then let go. They almost magically recoil and wind into each other, giving a hold as good as a knot, but our experience is that they don't work as well as laces and are more of a novelty.

Bathroom adaptations and aids

We had a lovely new bathroom fitted before I was diagnosed with MND, but the modern low-level toilet is so difficult to get up from. I don't want to spoil the look of the toilet just for myself, but is there any way of adapting it to make it more useable?

Old high-level toilets are much easier to sit down onto and to stand up from because there is less bending involved and your legs are more in line with your standing position. It is fairly easy to replace a toilet without major building work – the soil pipe and plumbing would probably be in approximately the right position for any toilet, but you can also purchase a sit-on toilet seat extension, a bit like a booster seat, that raises the seat by between 10 and 15 cm (4 and 6 inches). The extension has a lip that sits securely inside the existing seat, so it is safe but easy to remove so that other members of the family can use the toilet. Good chemists or medical supplies shops, or a disability advice centre, will be able to provide one for you.

I don't seem to have the dexterity or flexibility that I used to have and I'm not able to reach and turn to clean myself properly after using the toilet. Have you any advice?

Most of us seem to have been taught to reach around our backs to clean ourselves on the toilet, but you can probably do it more effectively by reaching between your legs. Remember though, that wiping toilet paper from back to front after having a bowel movement also can transfer bacteria from the rectum to the urethra. For this reason, women should always try to wipe front to back. This reduces the risk of bacterial infections like cystitis and urethritis. Also, if the toilet paper is usually kept on the cistern behind you, and difficult to reach, then move it to a wall-dispenser or somewhere else more conveniently placed. In places where the toilet paper is somewhere out of reach (like many public toilets) take a handful of paper before sitting down to save twisting or stretching when you need it.

If you still have problems, then you could try a portable or fixed washer for toileting. This basically consists of a small shower attachment to provide a hygienic wash, but you still have the problem of drying yourself afterwards.

How can I get my wife into and (more to the point) out of the bath? I used to be very fit, but I am over 70 now and I'm afraid of injuring her or myself if she slips.

Wet, soapy skin is indeed slippery on an enamel bath and it is easy to fall. Fortunately there are plenty of devices to help your

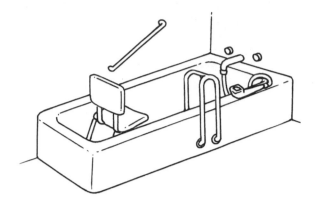

Figure 10.2 Bath aid.

wife as it is such a widespread difficulty. These range from simple aids for comfortable bathing to major structural renovation.

- A step could help her get into the bath, and she could also use it for sitting on outside the bath.

- A bath seat across the two sides of the bath or in the bottom of the bath would make it much easier for her to get in and out of the bath, or to wash her lower body without the need to get into the bath itself (Figure 10.2). Getting into (and out of) the bath becomes a two-stage process: from seated or from standing on the level to sitting on the bath seat, and then from sitting on the bath seat to sitting in the bath. Both stages are easier than climbing directly into the bath.

- A smooth-seated, backless chair or stool the same height as the bath can also be a good way to get into the bath – this will involve your wife sitting on the chair outside the bath, swinging her legs over the rim and into the bath and then climbing down into the bath.

- Handrails fixed to the walls at the ends and side of the bath provide extra support for getting in or out (Figure 10.2). These are just as useful in a shower cubicle, where support is essential when she has soapy feet on the smooth shower tray. The best arrangement is often two rails, one vertical and one horizontal, or one diagonally fitted rail to help her change from standing to sitting in the bath. Any rail used for support must be designed for the purpose. Towel rails and decorative rails are not strong enough and if they break with full weight on them, they are likely to cause more injury than if they were not there in the first place. A suitable rail must also be correctly fitted with bolts or deep screws to a surface that is strong enough to support them, and there should be clear floor space around them so that using the rail doesn't involve reaching, twisting or leaning.

- If the ceiling is strong enough – and this is vitally important – a trapeze or hoist can be fitted to the ceiling to give support directly over the bath where handrails can't be fitted. A motorized hoist takes all the strain of lifting your wife into and out of the bath, without any need to transfer her between seats.

- If you want to change the bath, then there are plenty of designs to suit people with mobility difficulties. These include (at the simplest) ordinary baths that have handles or grips on the two sides, baths with a built-in seat that would save your wife having to lower herself down to floor level, and (at the most complex) baths with a watertight door in the side.

- One other choice is to replace the bath with a shower – this will usually take up less space and involve much the same plumbing, so it should not involve any major structural work on the bathroom. A large shower tray fitted with a firm seat and a handheld shower spray is very convenient.

Can you give advice to help my husband keep some dignity and be able to bath himself as much as possible?

There are useful items available that aren't necessarily just for people with mobility problems:

- In the bath, a bath rack for shampoo or soap (and a good hook) saves reaching for everything.

- A handheld shower is a great help for washing and many wall-mounted showers are easily replaced with a hand-held hose and spray.

- A long-handled back brush saves a lot of reaching and your husband could wrap a flannel around it (or a small towel, if the flannel is too small) for soaping and rinsing his back, legs and feet.

- A non-slip rubber mat in the bath (the type that has little suckers on the underside) makes sitting up or standing in the bath much safer. A non-slip surface outside the bath is just as important – use wooden duckboards or a washable, non-slip mat on the floor.

Eating and drinking

I know it's not very sophisticated but I have started using a baby beaker for tea and coffee at home, so that I can actually drink it rather than spilling it, but I wonder what I can do if I have visitors or want to drink outside home.

You could take the bullish approach and just let people think what they like. If so, then have a look at the many stylish sports drinks bottles around. Cyclists, rock-climbers and campers all use adapted 'baby bottles' with sealable spouts for drinking on the move. Many camping and sports shops sell such bottles, in a range of materials including plastic, aluminium and steel. They can be difficult to wash, so they might not all be suitable for tea or other drinks that stain. Water bottles with this design are on sale everywhere.

Apart from that, there are many designs of cup and mug that are easier to handle than a teacup and saucer. A good design will be just heavy enough not to tip, have more weight at the base than in the sides and have a comfortable rim for drinking. There are some conical designs with a narrower neck than base, which are less liable to spills, but do need to be tipped further when you are drinking. If you have difficulty because of problems with swallowing, your speech therapist will be able to help and advise you. An occupational therapist will be able to advise on techniques that make eating and drinking easier, as well as equipment and adaptations that will help.

Some equipment is available on loan, although this is a fairly limited resource. Disabled Living Centres (DLCs) and the Disabled Living Foundation (see Appendix 2 for addresses) provide impartial advice and expertise on a range of equipment to help people purchasing specialized eating and drinking utensils as well as a broad range of other equipment. Local centres can be located through the Disabled Living Centre Council. If you want items that are functional but stylish, then designer cookware and tableware occasionally make an interesting, if haphazard, contribution, whilst cycling, hiking and camping gear is often both functional and stylish, although often a touch expensive. There are also some specialized shops if you have a very specific need in mind (e.g. Anything Left-Handed for left-handed versions of almost every utensil or tool you could imagine – see Appendix 2 for contact details).

My husband has great difficulty handling our usual cutlery. How can I make eating easier for my husband?

The right cutlery and crockery is important and it is amazing how impractical some tableware actually is. Often, plates are too flat to hold any liquid, cutlery too thin to grip or too long to turn upwards comfortably, cups and glasses too heavy to lift or so light that they fall over with only a small knock. Cutlery should have a good, thick, solid handle that fits the palm of the hand, should be balanced around the top end of the handle and have a working end that works – a knife should cut, a spoon should hold liquid and a fork should stab and hold solids. Eating with a spoon instead of a fork is always very effective or sometimes it is easier to use a dessert fork to 'stab' food rather than using a dinner knife and fork. This can be less messy and lighter than using a spoon. A large deep plate, such as an Italian pasta dish or a paella dish, holds food well and provides a good, upturned lip for scooping food at the edge of the plate. Fortunately, there are many sources of practical, stylish tableware as well as many sources of adapted tableware for people with disabilities. Your occupational therapist will be able to advise you on suitable crockery and utensils, and to suggest suppliers. The Disabled Living Foundation and Disabled Living Centres offer free, impartial advice on various equipment and utensils (contact details in Appendix 2).

I have real problems drinking soup. Can you suggest some special cutlery for me?

If you want to enjoy the soup as it is, without modifying the way it is cooked or served (see Chapter 7 *Problems with swallowing and breathing*), then it is essential that you have crockery and cutlery to suit your eating. Traditional, shallow soup dishes are perhaps the least appropriate design and a straight-sided, deeper dish might make it easier to fill the spoon. The spoon itself should have a deep hollow (some spoons are surprisingly shallow) and a flat, wide handle that makes it easy to keep the spoonful of soup level.

Rest your elbow on the table, whatever the rights or wrongs of table manners, and be sure to sit so that the soup bowl is high up and close to your mouth, to minimize the distance and height that the full spoon has to travel. In the last resort, use children's cutlery, plastic spoons, drinking beakers or thick straws – you are at the table to enjoy the food, not to behave well.

Another alternative (and a very traditional one at that) is to drink your soup from a teacup or mug because this might be much more controllable than a bowl and spoon. You will probably find that soup should be served a bit cooler than tea or coffee, because of its higher specific heat capacity – soups hold more heat than water and can scald your mouth easily.

My wife and I used to really enjoy going out to eat. Although I can still manage to get out with her in my wheelchair, I do find eating in public an embarrassment. Can you help?

We fully sympathise with your problem here. Ask for lightweight cutlery like dessert forks and spoons, or there is no reason why you shouldn't take your own adapted cutlery with you. Also, you can discreetly ask the waiter to tell the chef to cut your food up into mouth-sized pieces. This ensures that the meal will still look presentable as no chef will serve unsightly food. It also saves your wife's food going cold while she helps you cut your own food up.

Be it ever so humble, there is no place like home.

Furniture

How can I arrange our house to make it safer and more comfortable for my wife, who has had MND for 2 years. She refuses to accept any change and everything looks lovely, but I am afraid of her falling and can see she gets exhausted keeping it this way.

It can be very difficult to come to terms with rearranging a house around health needs, but it does have to be done to some degree. Often, very little substantial change is necessary, but you will have to compromise with your wife over how much change you can make and how quickly. The rewards are great in the extra time and energy that you and your wife will have left over for other things without the drain of keeping your house the way it is now.

In terms of safety, it is important that all the routes that your wife uses around the house (between the bathroom and the living room or between the kitchen and the dining room for instance) are clear of obstructions and have safe sources of support where she needs them. Firm tables and sideboards free of clutter and ornaments, placed at strategic locations can provide a much-needed boost when walking. Floor surfaces should be flat and non-slip – removing loose rugs and small pieces of low-level furniture greatly add to safety. Most houses have one or more extension cables to appliances or hi-fi far away from a convenient socket and these should be rearranged to run under a carpet or over a doorframe, or the appliances should be relocated nearer to a socket.

Instead of inconveniently located lamp switches and radios that require your wife to reach or stoop and fiddle with the knobs, it is possible to buy a remote control socket adapter for low-power devices (not irons, kettles or heaters). These can be used from anywhere in the room to switch on lights or other appliances. She could, for instance, set the volume and tuning of the radio as she likes it and just switch it on and off at the mains using the remote control handset.

A small bag, like a bum-bag or the neck-string wallets that holidaymakers wear to hold money and passports, will keep both her hands free when she is carrying things around, such as the TV remote control or pair of glasses.

A high trolley or television table on castors is a great help when your wife is eating snacks, holding drinks and putting down all those essentials (TV guide, remote controls, glasses or a book) that would otherwise go under a chair or on the floor. A small bag on the side of the trolley or a chair makes a good permanent home for those things that are always getting lost, like glasses. If your wife uses a neck-strap for her glasses, it is a good idea to keep it quite short, to avoid the risk of snagging the glasses on the table edge or other pieces of furniture when she straightens up or stands.

11
Care and services

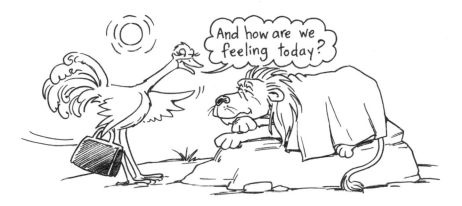

Caring for someone with MND can require a wide range of services. The amount and types of care will differ between any two people with MND according to the precise diagnosis, symptoms and personal circumstances.

I live alone and have just been diagnosed with MND. The GP gave me a thorough leaflet that lists physiotherapists, speech therapists, occupational therapists, just for starters. How do I go about contacting all these people and obtaining their help when I come to needing it?

You are unlikely to need to do very much yourself in the way of locating and making contact with medical professionals. The health service is very effective at providing the services that people need. Your first key contact is your own GP and, possibly, a practice nurse if your GP is in a group practice. Over time, and depending on your own needs, you may find that you deal more often with a community care worker, a community nurse or a social worker. In Scotland, an MND Care Adviser or MND Clinical Specialist coordinate other health professionals. Who you see will depend on the range of services that you require in managing your symptoms, caring for yourself in the home and staying active outside the home. It also depends on where you live and which services are available in your locality – unfortunately, there are regional and local differences in the availability of community care, what is sometimes referred to as a 'postcode lottery'.

> **Let the patient be in charge.**

Who is entitled to free treatment under the NHS? Am I going to have to pay for specialist drugs or physiotherapy, for instance?

Everyone resident in the UK is entitled to the full level of treatment provided by the National Health Service, irrespective of their National Insurance record and contributions. That means that hospital outpatient and inpatient visits, neurological examinations and 'standard therapy' are all available to everyone. This includes physiotherapy, speech therapy and occupational therapy, but these facilities vary with geographical distribution and are easier to obtain in some regions than others.

Prescription medications are paid for at the usual prescription rate, unless you are over the age of 60 years, in which case prescriptions are free. People who are on Income Support or whose partner is on Income Support are entitled to free prescriptions, dental treatment and sight tests (but not free sight correction such as glasses). These services are also free for people on Disability Allowance and certain other benefits. If you do pay for your prescriptions and need either regular supplies of medicines or need a large number of medicines each time, then there are procedures to reduce costs, such as the prescription 'season ticket' – ask for details at your pharmacy or chemist. Note also that no alternative therapy or complementary medicines are available on prescription and you will have to pay the full price for any you use.

Not all drugs are available on prescription, and some drugs are available on prescription only in some NHS Trusts – again a 'postcode lottery' situation. This means that you might have to buy some medications privately if they are not approved by your own Trust.

I am finding it increasingly hard to cope with all the work involved in caring for my wife. Is there any way I could apply for a home help or meals-on-wheels to help me out?

You need to apply to your local Social Services Department as your wife's primary carer or as someone involved in her care on a regular basis. They will then be able to conduct an assessment of your needs as a carer in order to provide you with the support you need to continue caring for your wife. If your wife's needs have not been assessed, then it is necessary to get this done first, because this may provide exactly the community care services that you want.

You can obtain further help and information from Carers UK (see Appendix 2 for details).

What is involved in a needs assessment?

A needs assessment is an evaluation of the community care needs of someone who requires assistance to remain in the community. It might be carried out by a social worker or by an occupational therapist working for the Social Services department of your local authority. The person carrying out the assessment will seek your views, as well as those of your GP and, possibly, of other people involved in your medical and day-to-day care. It is in your interests to discuss the care needs assessment with your GP beforehand, because your GP's influence is quite strong in the final recommendations. You might also be asked to complete a care needs questionnaire yourself, which you can do with the help of your GP or a carer if you wish.

Once your needs have been assessed, Social Services will plan out potential care with you and appoint a care manager to coordinate your care plan.

A care plan may include some combination of medical therapy, home helps of various kinds, laundry, meal services, odd-jobs, day- or night-sitting services, day centres or respite care. In practice, community care is dictated at least in part by budget and demand, so not all services are available in all places.

I am in the early stages of MND and hope to go abroad on a package holiday in Spain for 1 week with my wife. I am reasonably fit and active, but worry about whether I need to take any special precautions before travel?

If you are travelling in Europe, then there are a few particular things that you can deal with before leaving that can make life much easier if you do happen to need any kind of medical treatment while away.

First and foremost, make sure that you carry an adequate supply of all medications that you use. It can be difficult to obtain a prescription when away from home and some medications are simply unavailable in many countries because they are either not approved or not distributed. It is useful to keep the packaging and the patient advice leaflet that comes with any medication in case you need to describe the drug to a doctor or a customs officer.

There is an E111 European social insurance document that you can obtain from the Post Office or local government office. You can fill this in before travel to show that you are covered for certain medical care within the European Union. Buy adequate travel insurance before you travel and read the terms carefully, asking your agent to explain anything that you don't understand or that isn't absolutely clear. It is not very expensive and either payment or proof of medical insurance cover is required before treatment in many European countries – including even a simple visit to a general practitioner.

It may be helpful to obtain translations of key phrases,

particularly if you have any obvious symptoms that you might want to explain to people, such as difficulty in speaking or weakness in your legs or arms. Outside of the UK, MND is usually known as some variant of the scientific name 'amyotrophic lateral sclerosis'. For instance, in Spanish it is *la esclerosis lateral amiotrófica* or ELA. In French it is *la maladie de Charcot.*

Is there any way that my father could find someone to look after my mother on holiday, even for a weekend, so that he would be able to go away for a rest and a break?

Respite care is short-term or temporary care that allows a full-time carer to escape the non-stop, everyday worries of being responsible for someone else. Respite care may be overnight or may be for more extended periods of time. Respite is not a luxury, but an essential component of caring that maintains the health of the carer and reduces the risk of neglect and abuse. Nobody, no matter how loving or devoted, can care for another person 24 hours a day, 7 days a week, without risking their ability to care well or their own state of physical and mental health. However, respite care is in great demand and will not necessarily be free or even available, depending on where you live and what your circumstances are. Some charity organizations either provide financial assistance towards respite care or fund respite care centres and holiday homes.

Carers should, ideally, have some time alone and in peace every day (perhaps half an hour when your mother is asleep, engaged in watching TV or when someone else is at home) and a day a week away from the responsibility of caring (perhaps at a club with friends or engaged in some hobby). Respite care allows for longer breaks of a night, a weekend or a full holiday. Most employers, healthcare agencies and respite care centres would recommend that everybody has at least 2 weeks of care-free time in a year, and they aren't even referring to full-time home carers. Information about respite care and holiday centres is available from the MNDA/SMNDA and also the Winged Fellowship Trust, which maintains and staffs a number of holiday care centres throughout the UK (see Appendix 2 for details).

12
Employment issues

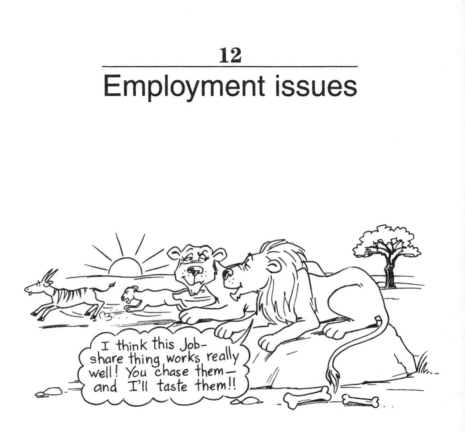

If you were still working when your diagnosis was made, you will probably have many questions about what you should and should not tell your employers or work colleagues, and what your rights are, especially when you become more disabled. Most of us never consider these issues until we actually need to and the complexities can be bewildering and frightening. We hope most of these fears are answered in this chapter. Most of the issues are actually fairly simple, so long as you know what it is you want and where to go for help and information.

Rights and obligations

I have been diagnosed with MND recently. Do I have to tell my employer and my colleagues once I have been diagnosed with MND?

No, you do not have to tell an existing employer if you do not wish to. At some point it is likely that you will have to explain absences taken for medical care or symptoms that affect your ability to do your job. When you choose to do so and how you choose to break the news is up to you.

There are advantages to telling your employer and colleagues about your condition, as well as disadvantages, and it is not possible for us to advise which course of action would be best in your own particular circumstances.

I had thought of changing jobs, but have now been told that I have MND. Should I tell future employers when I go for an interview for a new job?

If you attend an interview for a job, then you have an obligation to tell your prospective employers any facts that they ask for, which might be relevant to the employment. MND is almost definitely relevant because your abilities will undoubtedly change and you would be aware of this fact at the time of interview. If your failure to disclose information is subsequently discovered, then the consequences could be very severe for you, including dismissal and loss of some benefit rights.

Is there any way of making sure that my employer knows about my MND, but without having to tell all of my colleagues as well?

If you have an occupational health officer or occupational nurse, then that individual should not disclose information given in confidence, so you should be able to have your condition noted without everyone around you discovering your diagnosis. This could be very important, perhaps a lifesaver, if you were ever to suffer from an accident or dangerous incident at work and given emergency treatment.

Between yourself and your immediate supervisor (or head of department) it is likely to be a matter of trust that information you have given in confidence will be preserved in confidence. If you ask your supervisor not to disclose such information (explanations of absences, for instance), then that confidence should be preserved. Between yourself and your supervisor, it may be necessary to provide some explanation for colleagues, especially if you work in an environment where colleagues gossip. In addition, if colleagues suspect that you are unwell, they may have natural concerns that you have a potentially infectious illness. It might be helpful, for your own benefit as well as theirs, to provide some explanation of your illness in order to allay their concerns.

Do my employers have the right to sack me or make me redundant when they find out that I have MND?

Your employers cannot sack you because they become aware of your diagnosis. They can only sack you if there are material changes to your ability to perform your job adequately. In other words, if you need to take time off for illness or medical treatment, or if your symptoms make it impossible for you to do your job, then you will have to take sick leave according to the terms of employment of your job. This should specify durations of illness that are permissible and what procedures will be followed to terminate employment when employees are no longer able to work. You may consult a union representative (if you belong to a union at work) or the Citizens Advice can explain any terms of employment that are unclear. They will also be able to explain the statutory provisions of the law, if your particular situation is not covered or if you do not have a contract and terms of employment.

If you do not have a permanent position, there is little you can do if your employer dismisses you when your existing terms of employment come to an end, unless you can demonstrate that your diagnosis was the principal factor motivating your employer's decision, and also that the condition has no effect on your ability to do your job adequately.

So, the degree of legal protection that you have depends principally on whether you have a contract of employment, whether you are part-time (15 hours or less per week) or full-time, and whether you have worked in the same position for 2 years or more.

Is there any legislation to protect me and other people who are disabled from unfair employment discrimination?

There is a relatively new law, the Disability Discrimination Act 1995, that is intended to provide employment protection to people who are disabled. The Act covers obtaining employment, retaining employment and progression in a job. The Act prohibits employers from unjustifiably treating a disabled person differently from other employees for reasons related to that person's disability. In addition, the Act does not apply to certain categories of casual labour and trainees, nor does it apply to employees of companies employing less than 15 people.

If you feel that your employer is discriminating against you because of MND, but that you are still able to perform your job adequately (or would be able to do so with the support of your employer and reasonable adaptation of your working environment), then you may have a case under the Act. Because the Act is relatively new, it means that many of its wide-ranging provisions have not yet been tested in the law courts, but there is evidence that many employers are complying with the spirit of it.

My husband was exposed to hydraulic fluid for many years and we think it was this exposure that caused his MND. My husband doesn't want to create any bad feeling with the company, but I would like to know when and if I should seek compensation.

There are two questions here. The first is whether you should pursue your husband's former employer when your husband doesn't wish to do so. This depends on your relationship with each other and on how strongly he feels about the issue. If you did decide to take action, then it would be far better to do so with your husband's agreement and participation because his first-hand evidence would carry great weight.

If you are intent on pursuing compensation then the correct procedure is to find a qualified professional advisor with experience of compensation claims; your first choices are likely to be a union representative or a solicitor. They will need to find documentary evidence of exposure, your husband's illness and any previous illness that might be relevant (for instance, any evidence that symptoms preceded exposure would weaken the case) and scientific evidence that the exposure causes MND. They may also need evidence that the company was negligent, for instance in not providing protective clothing.

Before proceeding with legal action, bear in mind that no action has yet been successful in claiming compensation for MND. Given the current level of scientific knowledge about the cause(s) of MND, there is unlikely to be a strong case. You would almost certainly spend a great deal of time, effort and money in pursuing liability through the courts and get no settlement at the end of it.

In the criminal courts, you would have to show beyond reasonable doubt that your husband's MND resulted from the injury or exposure and that the injury or exposure resulted from your employer's action or negligence – in other words, that his MND could not result from any other possible cause. In the civil courts, you would have to show, on the balance of probability, that your husband's MND resulted from the injury and that the injury or exposure resulted from his employer's action or negligence – in other words, that the exposure is more likely to be the cause of your husband's MND than any other possible cause.

It is always worth checking whether there are any insurance policies or other cover (your husband's own or his employer's) that you can claim under. An insurance claim can be settled without admission of liability or guilt and without any courtroom appearances. It is also worth putting his case to his employer before resorting to the law courts to reach a settlement. Whichever route you choose, it is wise to consult an impartial advisor such as the Citizens Advice and a solicitor to establish the strength of his case.

Working with MND

I am finding it harder to cope with my job, particularly with tiredness towards the end of the day. How soon will it be before I have to give up working?

Individual variability is so great in MND that it is impossible to say how soon any one person will be affected to a particular degree. Your neurologist or GP should be in a position to say, in very general terms, whether they expect your symptoms to worsen rapidly on the basis of your initial symptoms and progression to date. The past is the best available indicator of the future.

There are people who have worked for many, many years after diagnosis with MND. It is possible that if the progression of your MND has slowed or stabilized, then you will adapt quite quickly to working within the limitations that your symptoms impose on you.

Would it be right to ask if I can change my contract of employment so that I can spend more time on things I find easy and less time on physically demanding tasks?

You do not have any right (legally) to change your contract to fit in with your new status, but it is in your employer's interest to maximize your value in the workplace. Therefore, if there are physical tasks that are tiring for you and are reducing your ability to work efficiently, then it would be entirely sensible for your employer to modify your job to accommodate your abilities better. If you can plan out a more efficient use of your time, then it is probably best to do so before consulting your employer so that you present a positive proposal rather than a negative request. Colleagues, of course, will be affected by any changes in your work practices and have every right to protection within the terms of their own contracts – so the more people you can convince of your case for changes in working practices, the more likely your employer will be to agree.

Is it possible to ask my employer to modify my working environment so that, for instance, I don't need to bend so often or walk so far?

It is certainly possible and your employer should make reasonable provision for you. Indeed, under the Disability Discrimination Act, employers are obliged to provide a working environment that does not unreasonably discriminate against people with disabilities. Obviously the word 'reasonable' invites a degree of interpretation – for instance, a modification that is reasonable in a modern office building may be impossible in an historic building.

If you can suggest changes to your working environment that do not cost an unreasonable amount, do not interfere with your colleagues' ability to do their own work and do not damage the fabric of the building, then your employer should have no reason to reject them.

Are there any sources of financial assistance for either myself or for my employer for any aids or adaptations that would make work easier and keep me working for longer?

The employment service runs the Access to Work scheme in order to provide practical help and financial assistance for disabled people who work or want to work. The scheme will sometimes pay 100% of the costs of specialized equipment or adaptations that are needed because of disability. Further information about this scheme is available from your local Jobcentre and the Disability Employment Advisor. The scheme is described in leaflet DS4 (1/00), called *Access to Work – information for disabled people*.

The Disability Alliance publishes a guide to public and private grants for people in need that contains details and contact information on many sources of finance, some of which will be relevant to your circumstances: *A Guide to Grants for Individuals in Need* (see Appendices 1 and 2 for details).

My colleagues keep doing things for me and covering for me at work. I know that they are trying to be helpful, but it is making me feel increasingly desperate about my own usefulness. What can I do?

Quite simply, you should tell them. They probably have every intention of helping you, as you suggest, and probably have no idea that you don't want this particular form of help. Of course, there may be an element of thought on their part (even subconsciously) that it is easier to do a task for you than to wait while you do it yourself. Either way, it will probably be best in the end to explain that you don't want this particular form of help. If you can suggest alternative ways that your colleagues can be helpful to you in your workplace, then suggest them at the same time, so that you make it clear that you are not rejecting their assistance outright.

Whatever you do, don't keep your desperation bottled up because it will lead to resentment of your colleagues, and ultimately they will have no idea what they have done wrong.

13

Financial and legal issues

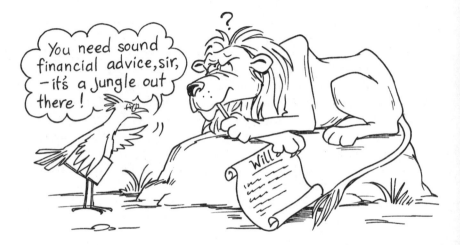

When someone has been the wage earner in the family, a diagnosis of MND can be frightening. There is help out there for both yourself and your carer. In this chapter we discuss financial help that will be available to you; what to do about the financial side of owning your own home; difficulties that you might encounter when trying to get insurance, and finally the more difficult subject of making a will.

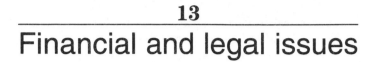

Anticipate the added financial burden.

Benefits

I gave up my full-time job when I was diagnosed with MND and when I thought I wouldn't be able to work much longer. Are there any benefits I can claim now?

It is very important to assess which benefits you are entitled to and not miss out on benefits you hadn't realized you were entitled to, both now and for the future. Benefits can entitle you to certain other services that are normally paid for – for instance eye tests, dental care, prescriptions and travel to medical appointments – and it can be well worth applying for benefit at an early stage to ensure that you will be eligible for these other services if you should come to need them. All benefit applications begin in the local Employment Service office or Jobcentre, where the staff will be able to tell you which benefits you are eligible for now, which you can apply for and what assessments might be made.

What benefits do you think I could be eligible for?

If you are not working and meet certain criteria you may be eligible for the *Jobseekers Allowance*, which many eligible people never claim. The *Disability Living Allowance* (under the age of 65 years) or the *Attendance Allowance* (over the age of 65 years) are for people who require personal care or supervision, or assistance with mobility. If you are unable to work owing to illness or injury (whether from MND or any other cause), and you have made sufficient National Insurance contributions, then you may qualify for *Incapacity Benefit.*

If you work at least 16 hours per week and have one child or more, then you can apply for *Family Credit*, which will be assessed on the basis of household income. If you are already claiming any incapacity or disability benefit, then you may qualify for *Disability Working Allowance.*

Whether you are working or not, you may qualify for *Housing Benefit* towards the cost of your rent outgoings. If you are severely disabled, then you may qualify for *Severe Disablement Allowance.*

Whom do I contact about receiving benefits?

You can find out about benefit entitlements from several places and do not need to pay for benefit advice or provide any details about yourself first. Sources of information include:

- the Post Office, which displays benefit advice leaflets for some of the most frequently claimed benefits;

- Citizens Advice which, in addition to stocking a wide range of leaflets and handbooks, are able to provide impartial advice on specific issues about your own situation;

- Social Security and Employment Service offices, which stock all relevant claim forms, and can help you to fill them in and ensure that you find out about all relevant benefits;

- your own local authority who will be able to advise you on services and facilities available in your own area;

- the *Disability Rights Handbook*, published by the Disability Alliance, detailed in Appendix 1;

- the MNDA or SMNDA with their nationwide network of advisors, detailed in Appendix 2;

- other charitable organizations and support groups active in your area who may advertise their presence through local library notice boards, in local telephone directories, in the local newspapers or at community centres.

Obviously, your final point of contact will be the Social Security offices, where you will have to register, complete the forms and apply for benefit. However, you may want to do some homework and investigation of the benefits available and the consequences of applying for them beforehand to make the process as painless as possible.

Is my wife entitled to any compensation for loss of income whilst caring for me?

No, your wife is not entitled to compensation for loss of income because of your illness. She may be entitled to a *Carer's Allowance* and this is independent of any income that she would otherwise be earning if she were not caring for you.

Home ownership

I own my house and have been told that I won't qualify for benefits. Is this true?

The equity invested in a property is counted as savings for the purposes of means testing, whether the property is your sole primary residence or not. If you are a homeowner or have substantial savings, you will be disqualified from receiving most means-tested benefits.

Can I give my home away to my children and then claim?

In principle and in practice, yes you can, but it is a high-risk strategy that is not recommended. It is also important to note that the value of your home is not counted as savings for the first 12 weeks of home nursing care or permanent residential care. The value of your home is also disregarded if it is occupied by a dependent (someone over the age of 60, under the age of 16, or receiving incapacity benefit) or, with discretion, by someone who gave up their own home in order to be your carer.

If you own your home outright and have no debts, then you can give your home to anyone you choose. If your total estate exceeds £250,000 (including your property and all other assets such as savings or shares), then it is possible, but not certain, that this action would be accepted as prudent tax planning. If your total estate is smaller than this, then it is likely that your property would be included in an assessment of your means. You could, if it is appropriate, either rent it back from them or include a clause granting a right of residence; in both cases this would eliminate the equity from assessment of your means. Of course, it will no longer be your property and you will have no control over it, nor any right to undo the arrangement if things improve financially at a later date. It is therefore absolutely essential that you make any such arrangement with the full knowledge of family members and others whose judgement you trust, and that all arrangements are contracted through a reputable law firm. Note that capital gains taxes will be payable by whomever you give property, savings or other assets to and that they will have to declare them to the Inland Revenue, so you may also need advice from a reputable accountant to minimize these costs.

If you do not own your home outright, then any change in ownership will have to be handled with your mortgage lender and this could be much more problematic. In practice many mortgage lenders are very eager to assist borrowers who have established a good record of payment. If you have had your mortgage for some years, then they should be willing to assist you. One possibility would be to transfer beneficial ownership of the fully paid mortgage to your child or children, or (if funds are available) to pay off the mortgage completely – in which case you can then do as you please with the property. Note as above, that transactions like these can be costly and are not easily reversible (and are indeed irreversible if the other party refuses to undo a legally binding contract), so sound legal and financial advice are both essential.

A further option for home owners, called 'equity release', is gradually appearing amongst banks and other mortgage lenders. It is a form of borrowing for home owners, which gradually reverts ownership of the property back to the lender as you borrow more from them. This can include an option of renting the property back from the lender. These equity release schemes are designed in particular to allow older people to enjoy the asset that they have spent a lifetime building without either selling up or living in financial discomfort when their incomes or pensions are no longer sufficient for their needs. A similar scheme exists to fund permanent residential care in the form of a 'deferred payment agreement', in which the local authority will receive payment out of the proceeds of property at a future date.

Insurance

I have had problems getting insurance. Do insurance companies discriminate against people with MND?

This depends what you mean by 'discriminate'. Legally, an insurance company is entitled to all relevant information from you before entering into a contract to insure you. Relevance here means any item of information that will help them assess more accurately whether you are likely to make claims under that contract at a later date. In the case of life and health insurance, this would mean telling them about your diagnosis and any test results you have had. Remember that at this stage you are asking for the best possible policy and nothing that you tell them can invalidate a later claim, but anything you know but don't tell them might do. The three possible outcomes of information that you disclose are that the insurance company will refuse to insure you at all; it could raise the cost of any cover offered; or it could reduce the quality or size of any cover.

Unfortunately, a diagnosis of chronic disease is likely to affect not just life and health insurance, where it is quite clear that your MND is relevant, but also car insurance, household contents insurance and holiday insurance, where it is less clear how MND is relevant to assessing future claims.

Insurance companies may not discriminate between people (i.e. treat them differently according to some characteristics) but are free to differentiate risk (i.e. identify individuals or groups of individuals who historically cost more in claims).

Any differences between a policy offered to you and one offered to another person in identical circumstances but without a diagnosis of MND are attributable to either an actuarial judgement of the increased cost of insuring people with MND, or to uninformed discrimination against people with MND. The first is legal and the second is not. Whilst it might seem unfair to people with MND, the insurance company does want to reduce the premiums for most of its customers in order to sell cheaper insurance. It can do so by levying higher charges on people who are likely to make greater claims in the future. It is up to the insurance companies to demonstrate that this is a fair reason for your higher policy charges. You are free to challenge them about increased premiums.

Are insurance companies allowed to ask me to undergo genetic tests or for results of tests that I have had? Will that affect my young children?

Insurers cannot require you to undergo genetic tests of any kind, although some insurers might occasionally request a medical examination (excluding any genetic testing) conducted by your own GP or by a clinician of their own choice. This is a request, and you can refuse to be examined with the risk of the application for insurance being turned down.

If you have had any genetic tests, then you are obliged to reveal this when asked. All insurers ask a question about information that may be relevant to your insurance cover or future claims. Telling the insurer about tests that you have had can do little harm. Failing to disclose information that you know at this stage could invalidate future claims.

At present there is no genetic test 'for MND', although it is technically feasible to locate some genetic patterns associated with a higher risk of MND (e.g. the superoxide dismutase-1 or SOD1 allele associated with familial ALS, discussed in Chapter 2). In the future it will undoubtedly be possible to make a more accurate assessment of the risk of MND and other late onset conditions. This issue is therefore of great importance in the insurance industry and they are eager to formulate acceptable procedures now while testing is still rare.

What will happen if I re-insure myself or change insurer (rather than stay with my existing insurer)?

If you already have a policy and have been paying all premiums on time, you are insured under that policy according to the terms negotiated when you took out the policy. So long as you disclosed everything at the time, your policy is still valid, even though your circumstances have changed. If you take out a new policy now, after being diagnosed with MND, your risk will be assessed accordingly and your premiums will be raised accordingly. It is therefore probable that your existing policy is better value than any new policy you would be offered.

It costs nothing to apply for insurance, and has no impact on your existing insurance, so do try to shop around for the best value. Remember that you must always disclose whether you have previously been turned down for insurance, and you should always keep your existing insurance up to date while shopping around for a new policy.

Wills

How do I specify who inherits what after my death?

Everyone should have a will. If you do not specify your wishes with regard to inheritance, your property and assets (your estate) will pass according to law to your nearest living relatives, normally a husband or wife for married couples, or divided amongst natural or adopted children when there is no marital partner. In the absence of a marital partner or children, the estate is divided amongst other living relatives. These rules are remarkably fair for the majority of cases of inheritance, but some cases cause much unhappiness. The usual pattern of inheritance can cause great distress and bitterness in many common situations including people married more than once, people with children by a previous partner, people with partners to whom they are not married and people estranged (but not divorced) from their former family. A last will and testament is essential in any of these cases (and many more not mentioned here) to ensure that your wishes are respected. Your will must be witnessed and signed and stored in a safe place where it can be found when needed. A will costs very little if you use a 'will kit', available from any good stationers or bookshop. A professionally drafted will from your solicitor costs more, but is customized exactly to your individual circumstances.

A will is also necessary when your estate exceeds inheritance tax thresholds and capital gains tax is payable on the excess. Payment of tax may require selling property, even the family home. It also surprises many people how much their estate is worth – the total value of the family home, all the savings, all property and lump sums payable on pensions and insurance policies can be much higher than many people realize. If this is true in your case, you should have your will drawn up by a solicitor.

Living wills

While I am still able, I want to choose how I will be cared for later on. If I write down my wishes and sign them, will they have any legal force?

A living will is an expression of your objectives and attitudes and does not carry any legal weight. Whereas many medical professionals will respect the content of a living will, they will only do so within 'reasonable limits' that will vary from one person to another. No living will can be obeyed where it contravenes the law or requires actions outside rules of professional ethical conduct. Members of the medical profession naturally wish to treat their patients to the best of their ability, and this may well conflict with your wishes.

A living will takes force only when you are no longer able to communicate your wishes yourself. Whilst you are able to communicate your wishes yourself, those wishes will take precedence over the living will. A living will typically lists your wishes in respect of life-saving and life-extending treatments and procedures. These might include your attitudes towards gastrostomy, mechanical ventilation or resuscitation (in the event that you stop breathing or your heart stops). A living will is not simply a list of things that you do not want, but may equally contain things you wish to emphasize that you do want.

In all cases, you need to discuss your living will with your medical carers and amend it where you agree with their suggestions. You may well need to rewrite it significantly after discussing it with them and discovering to what degree they will comply with your wishes. You may also need to rewrite your living will and discuss your views if you change medical advisors – for instance if you are transferred to another hospital, between wards in a hospital or to a nursing home or hospice – you may find the attitudes are completely different in different places. A pro-forma Living Will is available from the MNDA.

When it comes to it, I would rather not have any machine like a ventilator used to extend my life beyond the time that I can still breathe for myself. Can I refuse via a living will?

If you have strong feelings about assisted support, then it is vital to establish your views early on with both your family and your medical advisors. It is also vital to discuss any changes in attitude that you have as your symptoms change. Thoughts about your future will probably change as you face the reality of them.

In theory you can refuse any or all treatment. In practice, the circumstances in which a ventilator is first used are usually such that the patient is not able to express any opinion because you may well be unconscious at the time or in a state of emotional or physical distress. The establishment of a living will does make your refusal known, assuming that the individuals treating you at the time are the same medical advisors who were originally involved and have been made aware of the existence of your living will and its contents. A living will has no effect if nobody knows about it, and has greatest effect if you have discussed its contents with your doctors.

14
Coping with MND

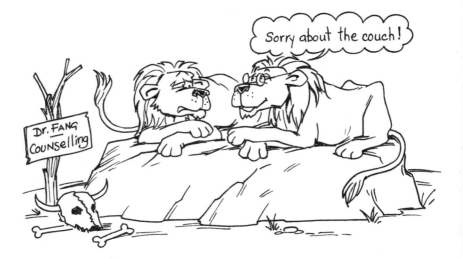

Life can be difficult enough with all the pressures of work, family and other commitments, without the added problem of MND. The impact of this disease is likely to point up both negative and positive aspects of your life before MND started, in work, family and relationships. Whatever mechanisms are used to cope, it is important to share the burden because nobody can cope alone. It is also important to recognize that your condition affects all the people around you as well as yourself – particularly partners, children or parents – and that they too will need support and understanding.

Coping as a parent with MND

How can I tell my children that I have MND and that I am not going to get better?

There is often very little difference between the emotional reactions of children and the emotional reaction of adults to the same circumstances, but there can be large differences in the expression of these emotions. Children are probably feeling very similarly to older members of the household, who often protect young children from difficult or complex situations, but even the very young are aware of the seriousness of the situation, even though they may not understand it. The big difference between children and adults faced with bad news is the way they react, the way they behave when unhappy and the way they express their feelings. Many children react to a tense or unhappy family environment with a sense of guilt, especially when they don't know the cause of the tension or unhappiness. Children may express themselves (depending on their age) through tantrums, bed-wetting, an intense preoccupation with other interests or freezing silence.

Children want honesty from their families and want to be included in family discussions. The more children are involved in discussions about your condition and treatment, the more they will come to understand without being presented suddenly with unexpectedly bad news. It is possible to be honest without divulging everything, for instance by focusing on all the care that is available and useful now, rather than on the progression of symptoms in the future. Hiding the truth behind an untruth is almost never a good idea because they will inevitably discover the truth at some point. At worst, your children may accidentally overhear a conversation or see correspondence or notes, and any untruths or partial truths that you tell them now may make them feel betrayed later.

Don't forget that some children may have very simple questions that they dare not ask, but which can be terribly upsetting for them. They might want to know, for instance, if they can catch what you have, or where they will live if you die, whether you will be better for their birthday or when you will next take them to their favourite place. All these questions need an honest answer, in as open a way as you feel appropriate. Above all, children need to feel that they are allowed to ask questions and should be encouraged to ask them.

Coping as the carer for someone with MND

I get so angry with my husband that he is no longer there for me, for the children or for our friends, and then I feel guilty for being so selfish. How can I cope better when I feel so bad?

Caring for someone else full-time is hard work, and caring for someone you have an intimate relationship with is doubly difficult – it may be that you have lost the largest source of companionship and support you had. Under any circumstances we all need to feel loved and appreciated, to have pleasure, enjoyment and companionship in our lives. There is nothing wrong with these feelings (it would probably be unusual not to have them), and guilt is a very common reaction to them amongst full-time care givers. Over time, the strain of caring for a partner or relative can cause stress and it is important to seek help and to care for yourself in order to continue. Symptoms of stress can include headaches, stomach ache, crying, irritability, disturbed or inadequate sleep and reduced appetite.

- Share your feelings of anger, frustration, inadequacy or being taken for granted – you are not by any means alone in having such feelings, and other people in similar situations can be a great help. Joining a local branch of the MNDA or SMNDA(see Appendix 2) is one way of meeting other families with MND.

- Take a break when you need it and spend time for yourself, whether actively doing something different that you enjoy or just relaxing and unwinding. There are often other people (parents, children, friends or neighbours) who would be willing to help out (perhaps by sitting in with your partner for a morning) but who you wouldn't have thought of asking – the worst that could happen is that they say no.

- Take care of yourself, your diet, your exercise and your sleep. If you feel the need to be vigilant overnight (e.g. because of your husband's breathing difficulties or because you have to turn him regularly) and you aren't getting any good nights of sleep, then see if you can ask someone else to help out one night a week.

- Pamper yourself, even if it is just with something small.

- Don't turn down all offers of help, don't try to do everything yourself and don't try to be a martyr – in the long run, you need to take care of yourself before you can care for anyone else.

- Maintain your social contacts and don't allow yourself to become isolated from your friends, relatives and the rest of the world.

- Maintain your family contacts, especially contacts that your children depend on for their identity and fulfilment.

A condition like MND puts tremendous strain on family relationships at exactly the time that those relationships are needed the most. Feeling that you are the primary or only carer and that you have no support is very difficult, so it is important that you do not try to cope alone – do look for help and companionship and accept it when it is offered. Nobody expects you to cope alone or to do everything yourself, and it is important for both of you that you accept the help you need to provide the care your husband needs.

> **Encourage positive thinking to heighten morale.**

Despair

I sometimes wonder whether there is a God at all, if he allows such diseases and pain. I used to believe there was and now I get very angry that I have MND.

A diagnosis of MND is a good reason for re-examining your spirituality and beliefs, or considering them for the first time. MND does force most people to consider their own mortality and beliefs about what happens next. For most of us, these issues are too intense and too complex to deal with on our own, and we need help to talk them through to a satisfactory resolution. Care is needed in choosing with whom to discuss your beliefs and how you raise the issues.

There are certainly a number of experienced individuals in every community who have the depth of spiritual resources and firmness of conviction to have been immensely helpful to others around them – for instance in helping others through the pain of bereavement, divorce or illness. If you have the fortune of knowing such a person well enough, then approaching them to talk may be a good starting point.

Formal religious advisors are there to help since it is their job, after all. There is marked reluctance to approach religious advisers or leaders in times of personal difficulty and reflection on their beliefs. If you have been a regular religious attender, then you will already know your advisors and their personality enough to ask for a discussion or to ask explicitly for help – don't be afraid to do so, because they are there to listen and talk. If you have not been a regular religious attender, then you will have the added difficulty of meeting your religious advisor for the first time but, again, do not be afraid. Most churches, mosques, synagogues and other places of worship are welcoming, hospitable places. If you are reluctant to attend uninvited (as most people are), then there is almost certainly someone in your circle of friends and acquaintances who does attend and would be more than pleased to introduce you.

People who do not have a strong commitment to a particular religion or denomination should not feel bound by their family background or cultural roots when choosing how to search for religious faith. If a group of people welcome you and provide the spiritual guidance and comfort you need, without asking anything in return, then don't be embarrassed to accept on the grounds of your difference in background.

One warning: don't allow yourself to become somebody else's charity project. If you are looking for spiritual reward, then seek it on your own terms and for your own benefit, rather than letting somebody impose their own needs on you.

There are some uplifting websites that you might like to look at (see *Appendices* for further details).

I am very afraid of dying. Will it be painful?

Many people with MND are afraid that they will be overcome by choking or swallowing difficulties and that they will suffocate, but this is not so. The most common cause of death for people with MND, as for everyone else, is respiratory insufficiency. This means a low level of circulating oxygen in the bloodstream from muscular weakness in the diaphragm. Death from respiratory failure or cardiac arrhythmia resulting from respiratory insufficiency is usually peaceful.

What comfort is there for my mother knowing that she is now going to outlive me?

When a loved one dies, it is common to feel a mixture of sadness, helplessness or numbness. It is also very common to feel a mixture of negative emotions including betrayal, anger, shame, guilt or fear. None of us can ever know how another individual will react to tragic events and, paradoxically, this is most true of the people closest and dearest to us. We therefore do not know how other people are going to react or what their needs are going to be unless we discuss it with them.

While some want to find out as much as possible, be prepared for every eventuality and find it helpful to talk about distressing things, possibly over and over again, others cherish privacy and silence.

You have the time to deal with these issues and the time to discuss them with your mother and family members. Sharing your experience and your mother's experience (if she wishes it) with others who have had similar experience can help. The MNDA/SMNDA and its members you have come to know are a good source of comfort and sharing. Another source is Cruse Bereavement Care, which offers free information and advice to anyone affected by a death. Cruse also offers one-to-one and group counselling. Contact details for the MNDA/SMNDA and Cruse are given in Appendix 2.

How can I help my friend with MND answer her question 'Why do I have to die'?

Although the exact cause of MND is unknown, it is safe to say that the onset results from a combination of nature and nurture, namely genetic composition and lifetime exposures. The condition is therefore down to chance and 'bad luck'. Nobody is selected or chosen to get MND and the condition is not a punishment for or a consequence of any sin or bad behaviour.

Most people want to know 'Why is it me rather than someone else?' and that is a question to which we do not yet know the answer. However, when you are helping someone through this difficult time, the points in the box might be helpful aspects for listening and discussing the issue of 'why'.

There has been a flurry in the media recently about assisted suicide. I sometimes have really black days and dream of 'ending it all'. I feel guilty about these feelings, but could someone help me to do just this?

There are many people who go through this – not just people with MND. Cancer, depression and many other conditions will at some point bring a person to real 'lows' in their life with resultant

How to listen and discuss difficult questions with friends with MND

Do:

- show that you are genuinely concerned, aware of their anguish and that you care;
- be available to listen, or be with your friend, or help with whatever seems important (no matter how unimportant it seems to you);
- let your friend talk as much and as often as needed;
- let your friend express unhappiness, anger, bitterness or any other emotion they want to share;
- be patient and encourage them to be patient with themselves;
- reassure them that it is not their fault.

Don't:

- allow your own sense of grief, anguish or helplessness prevent you helping your friend;
- avoid them because you are uncomfortable;
- say that you know how they feel;
- tell them what they should feel, think or do; or tell them to pull themselves together;
- change the subject to avoid discussing difficult or painful subjects;
- avoid talking about MND because you are frightened of reminding them – they won't have forgotten or put it out of their minds;
- try too hard to find positive sides to everything, or remind them of things to be grateful for;
- make comments suggesting that they are to blame for their MND or could have avoided it somehow, because they will have plenty of those thoughts, doubts and guilt of their own.

thoughts of suicide. If someone has a disease where suicide is not even an option, then the idea of 'assisted suicide' becomes almost an attraction. However, in the UK, this is illegal and, although the media has pointed out the choices of other countries where assisted suicide is now legal, you would still have to think about the consequences for the person you ask to assist you when he or she returns to the UK.

Changing relationships

Before my husband was diagnosed with MND our marriage was really on the rocks and we had decided to divorce. Now I feel really stuck because of his disability. We never let on to our relatives and I don't know what to do now. I feel so miserable.

At a rough guess, perhaps a third of all marriages are experiencing difficulties at any one point in time, although not all

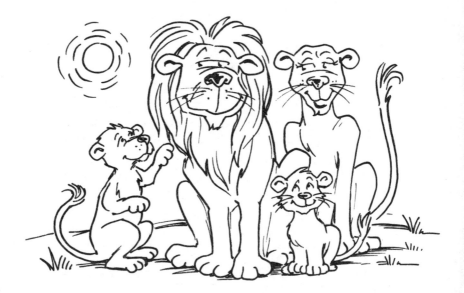

to the extent of being 'on the rocks'. Even so, you are not alone in having a diagnosis of MND coincide with or come after a marital breakdown. There is no easy answer as to whether you should stay with your husband or leave him now that he has been diagnosed with MND. If you stay, then there will probably be resentment and bitterness on both sides, but you will also probably be respected for it, and you will be able to support your husband in a time in your relationship of greatest emotional and physical need.

You have to assess what is best for both of you in the long run, including his future care and support and your future relationship with his family and others. The first stage is obviously to discuss your feelings of misery with your husband – you may find your relationship has changed greatly since your earlier discussions or arguments. Seeking help from a counsellor could help both of you.

All my freedom has been taken away from me since I was diagnosed with MND. I want to smoke but, as I am unable to get out of the house to buy cigarettes myself, and my wife says I shouldn't, I have lost this one pleasure.

Smoking is certainly not advisable, but then it isn't advisable for anyone, whether they have MND or not – but you knew that anyway. This is probably not just a question about smoking, but about a whole range of issues, and probably the central theme is your loss of independence. If you have not discussed this with your wife, then you certainly need to, because it is bound to affect every aspect of your life, from diet to clothing, even to what you do with your time. Try to find activities that both of you find acceptable and remember that compromise is probably necessary on both sides.

Having MND has changed the way people, even my family, look at me. I don't want people to feel sorry for me, just to take me as I am.

The best thing you can do is to tell them how you feel. They almost definitely have your best interests at heart and are not in any way attempting to belittle or humiliate you – although it can clearly feel like that when people seem to be sorry for you all the time. You need to make it clear that their pity, while well-intentioned, has very little practical value for you and does actually make you unhappy, uncomfortable or plain angry. If you don't tell them, then they will never know.

Remember that it is natural to feel sympathy and it is a part of the coping process when dealing with difficult issues. It is therefore important that you recognize that other people need to feel sympathy in order to cope with your illness (imagine how you might react if the roles were reversed) and it is important that you do not ignore their feelings totally. You need to come to some agreement on how their sympathy can be translated into actions that have some value to you.

I have mostly lost contact with all my acquaintances from work and am feeling very isolated from my former life. How can I go about making new friends and finding new things to do?

The key to meeting people is to be in places and doing things where you can meet. If you choose places and activities that like-minded people enjoy, then you are likely to make friends. Many have lives centred around employment and colleagues, so that they can become shut-off and isolated when they no longer work.

One possibility is to enrol in an adult education course of some kind. Adult education runs the whole spectrum from academic subjects like history, through more practical subjects like modern languages (e.g. Spanish or French), to art and hobbies. Many people discover talents that they never knew they had in water-colour painting, stained glass, pottery, carpentry and metalwork, for example. The range of courses on offer varies widely from place to place, but is generally broader in cities and near third-level colleges that have facilities available for adult education. The cost of an adult education course provided through local authorities is generally little more than the cost of materials and running costs.

Your family can also be a good, but untapped, source of company once you all recognize that your needs and your priorities have changed.

My husband was diagnosed with MND some months ago and it seems that we never make love nowadays. I miss this close relationship that we used to have. Is it that he can't make love now?

It is conceivable that your husband feels he is unable to make love because of his disease and how it has affected every area of his life. He probably feels diffident about discussing this whole aspect with you but it is well worth spending time with him and letting him know that you still love him and still want to have sex with him. In MND there is no loss of sensation in any area, unlike other neurological diseases such as multiple sclerosis, so there is no reason not to have sex. Indeed, it is to be encouraged as this is one of the best exercises around! You should try and continue to make love to your husband for as long as possible.

15

Future research into cures and causes

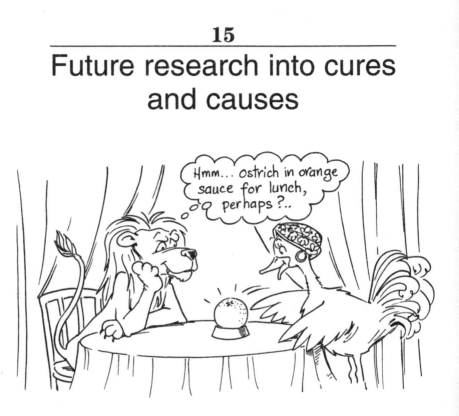

Throughout the developed world, people are living longer. As a consequence, degenerative diseases of the nervous system are coming to the fore. These include Alzheimer's disease, Parkinson's disease and MND. There is therefore increased funding for research in all neuroscience centres – it is difficult for any one person to keep up with all the developments, some of which are exciting, provoking further leads.

Never let the patient feel abandoned and alone.

The future of treatment for people with MND probably lies in current research into the condition, although medical advances are often unexpected outcomes of unrelated research. Many drugs used in the treatment of MND symptoms were actually designed for other purposes (such as the treatment of depression), but have useful side effects (such as a dry mouth). Here we present some of the research that was ongoing at the time of writing – there will clearly be new research by the time you read this, but the basic areas of research are not likely to have changed.

The newspapers are always printing stories about 'the cure' for MND, but none of them seems to result in any new treatments. Are scientists really close to finding a cure or not?

Science is moving apace and of course there is always a possibility of a breakthrough. These tend to be sudden and unexpected, so in one sense a cure could be close. That breakthrough may come from one of the many steadfast and relentless programmes of research on MND, or indeed as an unexpected outcome of other research.

Unfortunately, it is in the interests of scientists (who require funding to do their research) and journalists (who are in the business of selling newspapers) to make science stories more definite, more simple and more exciting than they really are. This means that stories that are genuinely interesting and important can get turned into apparent claims of a cure. The full story about a new 'wonder drug' may actually concern some species of genetically manipulated mice, where the drug has a small effect in slowing neurological damage, but the researchers don't yet understand the mechanism, the results may not be replicable in humans and all the mice suffered severe toxic side effects.

Surely by now, with all the funding and effort spent on research, the scientists should have found out what causes MND?

Unfortunately, progress is one thing that cannot be planned, organized or bought. Spending more money or time, or employing more people researching MND, increases the opportunity that important results will occur, but progress in research is often dependent upon chance findings and coincidences. The antihypertensive drug minoxidil, for example, was found to slow or reverse hair loss among people being treated for high blood pressure, purely as an accidental side effect. After clinical trials as a treatment for hair loss, minoxidil-based products are now amongst the leading treatments for baldness, but this is the result of a fortunate accident and not a result of any research into hair loss.

In the case of MND, a great deal is already known about the cells involved and how cells degenerate and die. This body of knowledge is continuously growing, and occasionally research findings do result in practical advances in the treatment of MND symptoms.

Do you think there will ever be a cure for MND?

A cure for MND, in the sense of totally reversing all damage in the central nervous system, would be a remarkable achievement. There is research using stem cells, which are cells that have not 'become' a particular kind of cell (such as a nerve or a skin cell), and it seems that some degree of nervous system repair may become possible. It is likely that such research will take many years or even decades to achieve significant results and there is controversy as to whether such research should continue. It would be an unwise scientific researcher to say that some development is impossible, but it is likely that local repair (such as recovering sensation from severed nerves in injured limbs) will be the first stage of what is possible.

New drugs for MND are being continuously investigated (see below) and brought into use and these are increasingly able to slow the progression of the condition. There is no drug at present, either in use or in research laboratories, that has the potential to halt the progress of MND completely.

Can I find out about the latest research on the internet?

Yes, an internet search engine will provide a list of documents matching a search word or phrase. If you are unsure about how to use the internet, there are some books available in any good bookshop that will give you useful tips about how to glean the best websites.

Note that there is no quality control of documents on the world wide web, so your list of documents will contain a mixture of academic research documents, useful documents from newspapers or support groups and documents that are either irrelevant or without any foundation. It can take a while to determine whether websites are trustworthy or not and which are nonsense. We list some websites we believe are genuinely useful in Appendices 1 and 2.

Genetics

If geneticists actually do find the gene for MND, will it change the range or quality of treatment I get? Could it lead to a cure?

Developments over the last two decades, have led to very extensive insights into and knowledge of the human genome and the proteins produced by many of the genetic sequences within it; this means that individual proteins synthesized by genes associated with particular diseases can be recognized and analysed. With luck and patience, from the many thousands of candidate locations in the genetic code, proteins involved in the MND degenerative process will be recognized and new drugs developed from this knowledge.

There is likely to be more than one (and possibly as many as 15) different genes associated with MND in its different forms. The immense research effort in molecular genetics is able to link the genetic patterns that occur in people with MND to the proteins that the genes code for. Ultimately, this will lead to a far more detailed understanding of what goes wrong during the progression of MND, even what goes wrong before onset, with the possibility of developing better and more effective drugs.

At present, a cure for established MND is not likely because cells of the central nervous system (brain and spinal cord) do not divide and replicate – the nerve cells that we have as adults are the same ones we were born with – and the widespread nature of nerve degeneration makes it unlikely that recovery of function is possible. Drugs to slow or halt progression seem much more likely.

Research is a difficult process of long years and most 'breakthroughs' result from luck, so it is impossible to predict when any significant new treatment will become available.

New drugs

Research into drug therapy requires large numbers of people to be treated, often with an experimental drug produced in small volumes (and therefore at great expense), and followed up for many months or years. The expense of clinical drug trials is almost always borne by the drug development companies themselves and rarely by public research organizations or by governments. Many thousands of drugs and therapeutic compounds have been developed to treat all manner of conditions, tested for safety and are in clinical trial; it is possible that one or more of these, by chance, will be recognized as having a therapeutic effect in MND.

Are there any drugs being researched currently that might come onto the market soon?

There are four major areas of research that are likely to lead to new drugs for the treatment of MND: genetic factors, the oxidative stress process, glutamatergic toxicity to nerve cells and damage to neurofilament-related proteins.

Genetic research into familial ALS (see Chapter 2) has

identified a different form of a compound called copper-zinc superoxide dismutase, a 'scavenger of free-radicals'. Free radicals are extremely unstable charged particles that result from normal metabolism and, if not checked or eliminated from the body, cause damage to nerve and other cells. Laboratory experiments are being performed to identify copper-chelating agents and compounds that mimic the normal behaviour of copper-zinc superoxide dismutase that will bind together with copper from the body and help eliminate them. Antioxidants fight stress caused by free radicals and include the well-known vitamin E, but many others are being researched.

Antiglutamatergic agents include riluzole (Rilutek), which has shown positive effects in human clinical trials, as well as lamotrigine and gabapentin, which have not.

Neurotrophic ('nerve nourishing') factors include a wide range of naturally occurring compounds produced in our own bodies (called BDNF, CNTF and GDNF) and hold great promise because they are a part of the process that protects us against the toxic byproducts of metabolism. Neurotrophic factors have readily observed effects in laboratory experiments with animal and human cells – so far, these have not culminated in any effective therapy, but research continues with compounds that stimulate neurotrophic factor production.

See the box on pages 146–7 for drugs that have been through and those still undergoing clinical trials.

Clinical trials

I have been asked to take part in a clinical trial, but I am not sure what this is.

A clinical trial is a formal method of testing new drugs before they can be approved for use in treatment. Every drug with a pharmacological effect must undergo clinical trials and only some complementary or 'alternative' compounds without significant pharmacological effects escape the process. Clinical trials ensure that drugs are safe and effective.

RESEARCH FOR DRUGS IN MND

Clinical trials under way at the time of writing

- **Buspirone** is an anti-anxiety agent that has a high affinity for serotonin receptors and appears to either mimic or stimulate neurotrophic factors naturally produced by the body.

- **Celebrex (Celecoxib)** prevents the release of glutamate and reduces free radical activity, which damages nerve cells.

- **Co-Q10 enzyme** is a naturally occurring essential co-factor to energy metabolism that appears to have antioxidant qualities. Early trials were very small, but indicated a positive effect on motor neurone survival.

- **Creatine** is a compound that is naturally produced in the body and enhances the ability of cells to use energy. Athletes and bodybuilders have used creatine as a dietary supplement. It is well tolerated and trials will determine whether creatine preserves muscle strength in MND.

- **Minocycline** is an effective antibiotic that enters the central nervous system easily. It inhibits nitrous oxide synthase, which damages nerve cells.

- **Myotrophin (IGF-1 or insulin-like growth factor)** is a naturally occurring protein associated with injury processes, and seems to both help the survival of damaged motor neurones and speed recovery after injury to motor neurones. Earlier trials of IGF-1 had conflicting outcomes and ongoing trials should resolve whether the factor has any benefit in, and for which types of, MND.

- **NAALADase** blocks the release of glutamate associated with nerve cell degeneration.

- **Neotrofin** has shown some clinical benefit for people with Alzheimer's disease but not yet in MND. It works by regulating genes associated with nerve cell regrowth.

- **Neurodex (AVP-923)** is not being tested as a treatment for MND, but may inhibit the distressing symptoms of emotional lability in people with pseudobulbar MND.

- **Oxandrolone** is an anabolic steroid (body-building supplement) that may, in combination with conventional dietary advice, preserve both muscle mass and muscular strength.
- **Tamoxifen (Nolvadex)** is the most effective treatment available for breast cancer. A chance observation of a woman with both breast cancer and a diagnosis of MND led to a small-scale trial to determine whether the drug slows the progression of symptoms of MND.
- **TCH346** is a novel compound undergoing phase 2 trials for its clinical effects on people with possible, probable and definite MND.
- **Topiramate (Topamax)** is an anti-epileptic drug undergoing trials to determine if its action will slow the progression of MND.
- **Xaliproden** (formerly called Sanofi drug SR57746A) seems to boost the production of naturally occurring neurotrophic (nerve-nourishing) factors such as BDNF, CNTF and GDF. Alone and in combination with Rilutek, this drug appeared to slow the progression of symptoms associated with lung function. At present, however, the manufacturers have decided to withdraw their application for regulatory approval for treatment of MND, although they still offer it to participants who wish to continue a longer-term trial.

Compounds that have previously been through clinical trials and appear to offer no benefit in MND include the following:

- **BCAA**, or branched chain amino acids in full (and having trade names Leucine, Isoleucine and Valine), did not prove effective in clinical trials and there was some evidence that their use may actually shorten survival in MND.
- **BDNF** (brain-derived neurotrophic factor), **CNTF** (ciliary neurotrophic factor) and **GDNF** (glial-derived neurotrophic factor) are all naturally produced compounds that protect and nourish nerve cells. No studies have yet shown any benefit from supplementing the naturally occurring compound.
- **Neurontin** (also called gabapentin) is a drug designed for the treatment of seizures, although some trials have reported beneficial effects in people with MND. No increase in survival is noted, although people taking the drug do report feeling better.

Once a potential drug compound is identified in laboratory samples, in other plant or animal species or in folk remedies, the first clinical test establishes whether the drug is safe in humans and what dose has an effect. This is a phase 1 clinical trial and involves only a small number of participants. A phase 1 clinical trial does not determine whether a drug is effective.

A phase 2 clinical trial involves a larger number of people, and aims to establish the effectiveness of a drug and the range of useful doses. A phase 2 trial necessarily takes longer to conduct (perhaps 2 years) and may begin as many as 5 or 10 years after a promising compound is first identified.

The final phase of clinical testing involves very many people, often thousands, all of whom comply with strict criteria that define the target condition for which the drug may be effective. The outcome of a phase 3 clinical trial assesses, statistically, factors such as survival time and functional ability of people who take the active compound over those who do not. The group who do not take the active compound under test may be taking another drug known to have certain effects, or a 'placebo', which has no pharmacological effect. It may take a long time to recruit suitable people for a phase 3 clinical trial, especially in rare conditions like MND.

The complete process from the start of clinical testing to approval as a commercial drug is often about 12 years, so drugs may actually be well known long before they become available.

What exactly will I be asked to do? Will my health be likely to benefit if I do?

If you meet the 'eligibility criteria' for a trial that is currently recruiting patients, then yes, you can take part in a clinical trial. The eligibility criteria are the characteristics of the people and the range and severity of symptoms that the trial designers want to include in their trial. The eligibility criteria are designed to make the trial as likely as possible to show a statistically meaningful result. That means that the trial will be sure to detect any differences in symptoms brought about by the drug, and be sure that, if no effect is detected, then this will be a reasonably certain finding that the drug has no real benefit. Eligibility criteria might include:

- *Clinical history.* Some studies will require 'the right kind of MND'; for instance, a study of the effect of a drug on the speed of progression of motor weakness might require that all participants have experienced some degree of worsened symptoms over the past year.

- *Clinical status.* Meeting certain diagnostic criteria (e.g. definite or probable MND and diagnosed within the past 24 months) or other score-based criteria, such as muscle strength or lung capacity.

- *Exclusion criteria.* Some studies might exclude certain factors from the study, for instance a history of heart disease or diabetes where the effect of the drug being tested on the circulatory system is unknown. Other common exclusion criteria are current or recent pregnancy, cancer, kidney disease, depression or being too young or old. Other factors might include the duration since diagnosis, and (for women) use of contraception where the effect of the drug on pregnancy is unknown or known to be harmful.

- *Place of residence.* For instance, an American study might recruit participants only from North America (the USA or Canada) in order to minimize the cost.

- *Continued availability.* The researchers will want to recruit people who are available for the research, available to be evaluated on a regular basis and will continue to be available until the trial is completed – perhaps as much as 4 years from the start of the trial.

In terms of whether you would benefit from taking part, the answer is both yes and no. You will certainly benefit from the regular follow-up and testing that is usual for all participants in a clinical trial, and would therefore be likely to receive more supervision than usual. Also, most of the time we think of clinical trials as drug trials, but there are also clinical trials of new diagnostic tests and procedures that, if they are in any way useful, would be of benefit to all participants.

Keeping to clinical trials of new drugs, you would be unlikely to benefit from the drug itself for two reasons: the first is that most trials are placebo-controlled, in which two otherwise identical groups of participants receive either the drug under test or an inactive placebo pill. You are as likely to receive the inactive placebo as the active drug. This is to ensure that the effect of the drug is compared between two groups receiving identical treatment in all respects (including follow-up, medical treatment and pill-taking) except the active compound. The second reason is that, before any trial begins, there will probably be no clinically significant outcome – the great majority of all clinical trials for all drugs and for all conditions do not show any effect.

So why, you might ask, should anyone take part in any clinical trial? Firstly, if you do take part in a trial, you will probably receive better medical care in general. Secondly, if the trial is a success you would be one of the first to benefit. Thirdly, and most importantly, clinical trials are the only mechanism for testing new drugs for people and no drugs will come to market without the generosity and dedication of the people who take part in clinical trials.

Glossary

ALS (amyotrophic lateral sclerosis) One distinct form of motor neurone disease that results in progressive weakness of the limbs. Onset may be in the feet and legs or hands and arms. The first symptoms may be simple clumsiness, tripping or dropping things.

anterior horn cell The cells in the front part of the grey matter of the spinal cord that connects the upper motor neurones (connecting the brain to the spinal cord) and form the cell bodies of the lower motor neurones (connecting the spinal cord to individual muscles). The final destination of motor neurones are the nerves which provide the signal controlling muscle activity.

atrophy The progressive loss of muscle mass, or wasting, caused by a reduction in the number of muscle cells. It is one of the later symptoms of MND.

biopsy The removal of a small sample of living tissue, often using a fine needle inserted under local anaesthetic. Muscle biopsy is one of the commonest techniques used.

bulbar Relating to the spinal bulb, which includes the brain stem governing the motor functions of speech and swallowing.

catheter A flexible tube inserted through the urethra and into the bladder to drain urine.

computed tomography (also called CT or CAT) scan Uses a finely focused X-ray beam that rotates around the body to construct a sequence of detailed cross-sectional images of the brain or spinal cord.

consanguineous Related by blood – relatives such as natural parents, grandparents and their brothers and sisters. Aunts and uncles by marriage are not consanguineous relatives.

cycad The cycad, or sago palm, is the source of an edible flour used in Guam. It is produced by grinding the large, soft kernel of the cycad nut to make a flour for cooking. The sago palm may

151

be sold commercially as a decorative plant, and normal contact with it is harmless. The nut contains a toxin that must be removed by long soaking before consumption. Cycad flour is not used in any food products anywhere other than Guam.

diagnosis The process of establishing the origin of clinical symptoms and identifying the underlying pathology (disease) which is responsible for them. Neurological diagnosis can be a complex process of elimination of differential diagnoses because many identical neurological symptoms can have different underlying pathologies.

familial Approximately 5% of all cases of ALS are believed to be familial cases, occurring in clusters of families in which more than one individual in the family are affected. The onset of familial MND tends to be earlier than in sporadic MND with slower progression and longer survival.

fasciculation Irregular and involuntary contractions of muscle bundles, of variable frequency. The contractions are often visible across the shoulders and in the forearm. Whilst fasciculation is evidence for a diagnosis of MND, it may also result from other neurological diseases, and may be present in normal individuals.

gastrostomy The introduction of a feeding tube directly into the stomach through a small opening in the abdomen.

Guam An island in the Pacific in which a high-incidence focus of MND and Parkinsonism has been extensively researched. A number of prominent causative hypotheses have been inconclusively studied, including cycad poisoning and mineral deficiency.

ICD-9 The Ninth Revision of the International Classification of Disease provides a comprehensive coding system for use in classifying medical data. The broad (3-digit) code for MND is 335 (anterior horn cell disease), which includes the more specific (4-digit) codes 335.0 (Werdnig–Hoffman disease), 335.1 (spinal muscular atrophy), 335.2 (motor neurone disease), 335.8 (other types) and 335.9 (a residual category of unspecified types).

incidence The occurrence of new cases of a condition. The incidence rate describes the frequency with which cases are identified. Incidence is commonly measured in new cases per 1000 (or 100,000) of population at risk, per year. The incidence of MND typically varies between 1 and 4 new cases per 100,000 of population per year in Western nations and is much lower in developing nations, where life expectancy is shorter.

Kii Peninsula The Kii Peninsula of Japan, in which a high-incidence focus of MND has been observed. A number of hypotheses relating to mineral and metal deficiency and exposure have been put forward to explain the local excess but none has been confirmed.

Kugelberg–Welander disease Benign spinal muscular atrophy, a form of motor neurone disease with a juvenile onset and long course.

lability Liable to change, instability. Emotional lability is the sudden change of mood (euphoria, sadness, etc.) without any apparent triggering factors. It is a feature of pseudobulbar palsy.

laminectomy Partial or complete surgical removal of laminae (vertebral arches of the spinal column) to expose the spinal cord and obtain spinal cord decompression. The surgical operation is intended to relieve pressure on the spinal cord or nerve roots.

lumbar puncture The withdrawal of cerebrospinal fluid under local anaesthetic from the space below the spinal cord through a hollow needle inserted between the vertebrae of the spinal column in the lower back. The fluid, which surrounds the spinal cord and brain, may be examined for protein content, viral or bacterial infection, or the breakdown products of immune responses.

magnetic resonance imaging (also called MRI) scans Use of a strong magnetic field to induce resonating radio wave emission from hydrogen atoms in body tissue. Adjustments in these waves can be made to detect different types of tissue and, unlike X-rays, magnetic resonance does not depend on absorption by hard tissues (like bone) and so it can be used to image muscle and nervous system tissue in great detail.

medulla The medulla oblongata is the part of the brain stem connecting the brain to the spinal cord.

MND (motor neurone disease) Motor neurone diseases (or anterior horn cell diseases) include Werdnig–Hoffman disease (or infantile spinal muscular atrophy), spinal muscular atrophy (juvenile Kugelberg–Welander and adult forms), motor neurone disease (amyotrophic lateral sclerosis, progressive bulbar palsy and progressive muscular atrophy).

neurone (or neuron) A general term for nerve cells. The nerve cells of importance in MND are the upper motor neurones and the lower motor neurones; the anterior horn cells are the cell bodies of the latter.

NIPPV Non-invasive positive pressure ventilation (commonly known as a nippy).

onset The time of appearance of the first symptoms of a condition. Onset may actually precede the realization that anything is wrong, when there will be gradual changes in function.

PBP (progressive bulbar palsy) Progressive bulbar palsy, a form of MND resulting in difficulty in speech and swallowing with wasting and fibrillation (fasciculation) of the tongue.

percutaneous endoscopic gastrostomy Sometimes called a 'peg' for short.

PMA (primary muscular atrophy) Primary muscular atrophy, a form of MND in which the lower motor neurones only are affected.

prognosis The outlook, or considered probable course, for a patient.

pyramidal tract The tract of nerve fibres that consist of upper motor neurones and run from the brain to the anterior horn cells of the spinal cord.

SMA (spinal muscular atrophy) Spinal muscular atrophy or infantile spinal muscular atrophy (see also Werdnig–Hoffman's disease and Kugelberg–Welander disease)

SOD (superoxide dismutase) Superoxide dismutase is an enzyme that inactivates free radicals, protecting cells from damaging chemical reactions. The gene identified in familial ALS codes for this enzyme.

sporadic Occurring randomly, without any apparent pattern or cause. Approximately 95% of all cases of MND are sporadic, occurring in individuals with no familial history of the condition.

suprapubic Above the pubic bone. A suprapubic catheter is a catheter that is inserted through the abdominal wall instead of through the urethra to drain the bladder.

trachea The windpipe, which carries air down into the lungs.

tracheostomy A surgical opening into the trachea for the insertion of a tube to ease breathing difficulties.

Werdnig–Hoffman's disease Infantile spinal muscular atrophy.

Appendix 1
Books and other sources of information

Publications on MND and associated disorders

Amyotrophic Lateral Sclerosis: a guide for patients and families,
by Hiroshi Mitsumoto and Theodore L Munsat,
published by Demos Medical Publishing, New York, 2001,
ISBN 1 888 799285.

Amyotrophic Lateral Sclerosis, by Hiroshi Mitsumoto, David A Chard
and Erik P Pioro,
published by Oxford University Press, 1998, ISBN 0 803 602693.
Recommended for health professionals.

Disability Rights Handbook,
published by the Disability Alliance Education & Research Association.
This book is updated annually – the 27th edition was published in May
2002 – and is acknowledged as the most comprehensive reference guide
on social security benefits and services for disabled people. The
Handbook includes information on benefits in residential care and
hospital, industrial injuries provision, the rules around welfare to work
benefits, war pensions, a step-by-step guide to the appeals procedure
and benefits for carers, as well as sections on income tax and a
directory of essential addresses.

*MND Resource File: a patient and carer centred approach for health
and social care professionals,*
published by the MNDA, 2000 (purchase via the MNDA website only).

Motor Neuron Disease, edited by RW Kuncl,
published by WB Saunders, 2002, ISBN 0 702 025283.

Motor Neurone Disease: a family affair, by Dr David Oliver, published by Sheldon Press, 1995 ISBN 0 859 697053. Recommended for newly diagnosed patients.

Your Personal Guide to Motor Neurone Disease, published by the MNDA, 2002, (purchase via the MNDA only).

Websites and mailing lists on MND

There are many websites available on MND. Be wary of the information available as many can be misleading with hopes about miracle cures. The sites below have quality information. Remember that some of the best information can be obtained via the websites of the national associations (MNDA and SMNDA) and the international associations (e.g. ALSA) (see Appendix 2 for their addresses and website addresses).

ALS Digest
A helpful electronic mailing list set up to serve the needs of people with MND, their friends and families, researchers and medics involved with MND. Subscription to an email address is free.
www.alslinks.com/currentdigest.htm

ALS/MND Research Mail List
www.als-tdf.org/alstdf/research/hubben/signup.asp

ALS Research Therapy Foundation
www.als.net.alstdf
www.alslinks.com/alsdigestarchives.htm

Clinical trials summary from the NHS
www.clinicaltrials.gov

Research news
www.dukenews.duke.edu/research/regener.htm
www.nature.com/nsu/020819/020819-11.html
www.flinders.edu.au/news/articles/?fj20v12s01
www.sciencenews.org/sn_arch/9_21_96/fob1.htm
www.mcg.edu/news/mcgtomorrow/n5_mcclusky.htm

World Federation of Neurology, ALS page
www.wfnals.org

PALS (People with ALS)
http://home/goulburn/net/au~shack
Steven Shackel's website – a knowledgeable person with ALS, Steven
has won an award for Academic Excellence in Australia.

http://www.hopeforals.com/html/eedney.html
Eric Edney's website – an inspiring website.

SALSA (Supporting Amyotrophic Lateral Sclerosis Associates)
Jarrod Cunningham developed MND and together with his wife has set
up the charity SALSA. Their website is www.salsassociates.com (at present
in development). The charity is to be registered in mid-2003. A support
service is available on 020 8549 4937.

Search engines

Suitable search engines include Google (www.google.com), Microsoft-
Networks (www.search.msn.com), Altavista (www.altavista.com) and Infoseek
(www.infoseek.go.com), but there are many others and each will return
different results; www.omni.ac.uk is a good place to try for quality
websites. Remember to search for MND as well as amyotrophic lateral
sclerosis (ALS) or Lou Gehrig's disease.

You will also find a search facility on many newspaper websites (e.g.
The Guardian at www.guardian.co.uk) for news items appearing in
current and previous editions of the paper.

Other publications

The English Heritage Visitors Handbook,
published by English Heritage, Swindon, 2002 (updated regularly),
ISBN 1 850 748209 2002.
An invaluable guide for planning a day out in England, this book
contains up-to-date information on over 400 historic properties cared
for by English Heritage. Highly illustrated with full-colour photographs
and maps, the guide also lists all the historic sites in Scotland, Wales
and the Isle of Man. This book comes free with their Membership
Welcome Pack.

A Guide to Grants for Individuals in Need,
published by the Directory of Social Change, Liverpool/London, 2002
(updated regularly), ISBN 1 903 991250.

The National Trust Handbook,
published by the National Trust, London.
Published annually as a paperback or combined with membership.
Information for visitors with disabilities is available in print or for free
download: www.nationaltrust.org.uk/main/placestovisit/disability.pdf.
A substantial information booklet is available to view as an Adobe
Acrobat pdf file, or you can order a free printed copy in standard or
large print or on tape. It contains details of facilities available for
visitors with disabilities, as well as information about touch
opportunities at our properties and a list of National Trust holiday
cottages, which have been adapted for accompanied wheelchair users.
See Appendix 2 for address details.

RHS Garden Finder, by Charles Quest-Ritson,
published by Dorling Kindersley, London, 2003/2004 (updated
regularly), ISBN 0 751 364339.
An expanded version of the RHS Garden Finder, first devised for the
RHS website (search online), is now available in book form.
It describes over 1000 notable gardens and nurseries to visit in the UK.
An alphabetical listing of specialities – particular plants, National
Collections, historical interest – enables the reader to find gardens with
appropriate displays. Organized in county order, the book includes full
address and contact details, opening times, location map and facilities
offered for each garden as well as a description by the author.

Appendix 2
Useful addresses

MND associations

National

Motor Neurone Disease Association
PO Box 246
Northampton NN1 2PR
Helpline: 08457 626262
Tel: 01604 250505
Fax: 01604 638289
Website. www.mndassociation.org
Offers information and support to people with motor neurone disease and their families. Has local branches and funds medical research.

Scottish Motor Neurone Disease Association
76 Firhill Road
Glasgow G20 7BA
Tel: 0141 945 1077
Fax: 0141 945 2578
Website: www.scotmnd.org.uk
Offers information and support to people with motor neurone disease and their families. Has local branches and funds medical research.

International

ALS Association – National Office
27001 Agoura Road
Suite 150
Calabasas Hills
California CA 93101
USA
Tel: 00 1 818 880 9007
Fax: 00 1 818 880 9006
The ALS Association (ALSA) is the only national not-for-profit voluntary health organization dedicated solely to the fight against amyotrophic lateral sclerosis (often called Lou Gehrig disease). Aims to find a cure for and improve living with ALS.

**Irish Motor Neurone Disease
Association**
Coleraine House
Coleraine Street
Dublin 7
Eire
Tel: 00 353 1 8730422
Fax: 00 353 1 8731409
*Offers information and support
to people with motor neurone
disease and their families.*

**International Alliance of
ALS/MND Associations**
Website: alsmndalliance.org

Other MND-related organizations

**John Bevan MND Research
Unit**
Centre for the Study of Health,
Sickness and Disablement
(CSHSD)
Brunel University
Uxbridge UB8 3PH
Website:
www.brunel.ac.uk/research/cshsd/

**World Federation of
Neurology ALS/MND Group**
12 Chandos Street
London W1G 9DR
Tel: 020 7323 4011
Fax: 020 7323 4012
Website: www.wfneurology.org
*An international federation
monitoring neurological studies
worldwide.*

Other useful addresses

**3H Fund (Help the
Handicapped Holiday Fund)**
147a Camden Road
Tunbridge Wells TN1 2RA
Tel: 01892 547474
Fax: 01892 524703
Website: www.3hfund.org.uk
*Subsidized group holidays for
physically disabled children and
adults with volunteer carers,
offering respite for regular
carers. Grants to low income
families with physically or
mentally disabled dependents to
have a modest UK holiday.
Apply direct.*

Abilitynet
PO Box 94
Warwick CV34 5WS
Helpline: 0800 269545
Tel: 01926 312847
Fax: 01926 407425
Website: www.abilitynet.co.uk
*Advice and support to help make
the benefits of using computers
available to disabled children
and adults. Can arrange
assessment at home or in the
work place for a fee.*

Age Concern England
Astral House
1268 London Road
London SW16 4ER
Helpline: 0800 009966
Tel: 020 8765 7200
Fax: 020 8765 7211
Website: www.ageconcern.org.uk
*Researches into the needs of
older people and is involved in
policy making. Publishes many
books and has useful fact sheets
on a wide range of issues from
benefits to care, and provides
services via local branches.*

Age Concern Scotland
113 Rose Street
Edinburgh EH2 3DT
Helpline: 0800 009966
Tel: 0131 220 3345
Fax: 0131 220 2779
Website:
www.ageconcernscotland.org.uk
*Information sheets and local
support groups offering a
variety of services to the elderly.*

Anything Left-Handed
18 Avenue Road
Belmont, Surrey SM2 6JD
Tel: 020 8770 3722
Fax: 020 8715 1220
Website:
www.anythingleft-handed.co.uk
*Distributors of left-handed items
manufactured all over the world.
Shop and mail order catalogue.
Deliveries to all parts of the*
*globe. Custom-made items also
available.*

AREMCO
Grove House
Lenham
Kent ME17 2PX
Tel: 01622 858502
Fax: 01622 850532
*Supplier of a variety of
equipment, aids and tools for
people with disabilities;
protective headgear, bed-leaving
alarms and swivel seats for cars
etc.*

**Association of Community
Health Councils for England
and Wales**
Earlsmead House
30 Drayton Park
London N5 1PB
Tel: 020 7609 8405
Fax: 020 7700 1152
Website: www.achcew.org.uk
*Headquarters for local
community health councils who
represent the needs of the
patient.*

Association of Disabled Professionals
BCM ADP
London WC1N 3XX
Tel: 020 8778 5008
Fax: 020 8778 5008
Website: www.adp.org.uk
Promotes education, rehabilitation, training and employment opportunities available to professional people with disabilities. Offers advice, information and peer support to disabled people. Also funds research.

Benefits Agency
The address and telephone number of your local Benefits Agency will be in the Phone Book and in Yellow Pages under Social Services. Government agency with information and advice on all types of benefits. (See also Benefits Enquiry Line for people with disabilities.)

Benefits Enquiry Line (BEL) for people with disabilities
Freephone: 0800 882200
(England, Scotland and Wales)
Freephone: 0800 220674
(Northern Ireland)
Website: www.dwp.gov.uk
Minicom: 0800 243355
Government agency giving information and advice on benefits for people with disabilities.

British Association for Counselling and Psychotherapy
1 Regent Place
Rugby CV21 2PJ
Helpline: 0870 443 5252
Tel: 01788 550899
Fax: 0870 443 5160
Website: www.counselling.co.uk
Professional services organization and impartial register for counsellors. Offers lists of all levels of counsellors and can refer to specialist counselling services.

British Complementary Medicine Association
PO Box 5122
Bournemouth BH8 OWG
Tel: 0845 345 5977
Fax: 0845 345 5978
Website: www.bcma.co.uk
Multitherapy umbrella body representing organizations, clinics, colleges and independent schools, and acting as the voice of complementary medicine.

British Council of Disabled People
Litchurch Plaza
Litchurch Lane
Derby DE24 8AA
Tel: 01332 295551
Fax: 01332 295580
Minicom: 01332 295581
Website: www.bcodp.org.uk
Support for organizations of disabled people.

British Medical Acupuncture Society
12 Marbury House
Higher Whitley
Warrington WA4 4QW
Tel: 01925 730727
Fax: 01925 730492
Website:
www.medical-acupuncture.co.uk

British Red Cross Society
Website: www.redcross.org.uk
Provides equipment on loan, transport and escort services for which there is usually a small charge. Local branches are listed in the telephone directory.

British Society for Disability and Oral Health
Dental Special Needs Unit
Chorley District General Hospital
Preston Road
Chorley PR7 1PP
Tel. 01257 245664
Website: www.bsdh.org.uk
NHS dental service for people with disabilities with dental problems.

British Wheel of Yoga
25 Jermyn Street
Sleaford NG34 7RU
Tel: 01529 306851
Fax: 01529 303233
Website: www.bwy.org.uk
Professional body offering lists of qualified yoga therapists.

Carers UK
20–25 Glasshouse Yard
London EC1A 4JT
Helpline: 0808 808 7777
Tel: 020 7490 8818
Fax: 020 7490 8824
Website: www.carersonline.org.uk
Offers information and support to all people who have to care for others owing to medical or other problems.

Chivers Large Print Books
Chivers Press Ltd
Windsor Bridge Road
Bath BA2 3AX
Tel: 01225 335336
Fax: 01225 310771
Website:
www.audiobookcollection.com
Books in large print and audio tapes for sale. Mail order only.

Toby Churchill Ltd
20 Panton Streetg
Cambridge CB2 1HP
Tel: 01223 576117
Fax: 01223 576118
Website: www.toby-churchill.com
Provides communication aids and offers home assessment to people with special needs. Repair service.

Citizen Advocacy Information and Training (CAIT)
162 Lea Valley Technopark
Ashley Road
Tottenham Hale
London N17 9LN
Tel: 020 8880 4545
Fax: 020 8880 4113
Website: www.citizenadvocacy.org.uk
Promotes, supports and offers free, friendly advocacy by one citizen to another.

Citizens Advice
Myddleton House
115–123 Pentonville Road
London N1 9LZ
Helpline: 0870 750 9000
Tel: 020 7833 2181
Fax: 020 7833 4371
Website: www.citizensadvice.org.uk
and www.adviceguide.org.uk
Headquarters of national charity offering a wide variety of practical, financial and legal advice. Has a network of local branches throughout the UK. The address and telephone number of your local CAB will be in the Phone Book and in Yellow Pages under Counselling and Advice. National charity offering a wide variety of practical, financial and legal advice. Has local branches throughout the UK.

Citizens Advice Scotland
26 George Square
Edinburgh EH8 9LD
Tel: 0131 667 0156
Fax: 0131 668 4359
Website: www.cas.org.uk
Provide details of local Citizens Advice Bureaux, which are also available in local telephone directories.

Community Service Volunteers
237 Pentonville Road
London N1 9NJ
Tel: 020 7278 6601
Fax: 020 7833 0149
Website: www.csv.org.uk
Encourages people through training and support to take action in their communities. Provides volunteers to work full time in social care placements for periods of 4–12 months.

Continence Foundation
307 Hatton Square
16 Baldwins Gardens
London EC1N 7RJ
Helpline: 0845 345 0165
Tel: 020 7404 6875
Fax: 020 7404 6876
Website:
www.continence-foundation.org.uk
Offers information and support for people with bladder and/or bowel problems. Has lists of regional specialists.

Crossroads (Caring for Carers)
10 Regent Place
Rugby CV21 2PN
Tel: 0845 450 0350
Fax: 01788 565498
Provides short-term breaks to carers in their own homes.

Crossroads Scotland
24 George Square
Glasgow G2 1EG
Tel: 0141 226 3793
Fax: 0141 221 7130
Website:
www.crossroads-scotland.co.uk
Information leaflets and support for carers within own homes, for any age, disability and sickness. Local branches.

Cruse Bereavement Care
Cruse House
126 Sheen Road
Richmond TW9 1UR
Helpline: 0870 167 1677
Tel: 020 8939 9530
Fax: 020 8940 7638
Website:
www.crusebereavementcare.org.uk
Offers information, practical advice, sells literature and has local branches which can provide one-to-one counselling to people who have been bereaved. Training in bereavement counselling for professionals.

Department of Health
PO Box 777
London SE1 6XH
Tel: 020 7210 4850
Fax: 01623 724524
Website: www.doh.gov.uk
NHS information leaflets on alcohol, drugs, children and family, sexual health, immunization and older people. (Previously provided by Health Promotion, England.)

DIAL UK
St Catherines Hospital
Tickhill Road
Balby
Doncaster DN4 8QN
Tel: 01302 310123
Fax: 01302 310404
Website: www.dialuk.org.uk
Offers advice on all aspects of disability.

Disabilities Trust
First Floor
32 Market Place
Burgess Hill RH15 9NP
Tel: 01444 239123
Fax: 01444 244978
Website: www.disabilities-trust.org.uk
Offers care and long-term accommodation for people with autism, acquired brain injury and physical disabilities at 18 centres across England.

Disability Alliance
First Floor East
Universal House
88–94 Wentworth Street
London E1 7SA
Tel: 020 7247 8776
Fax: 020 7247 8765
Website: www.disabilityalliance.org
Publishes Disability Rights
Handbook *and* A Guide to Grants
for Individuals in Need. *Authority
on social security benefits for
people with disability.*

**Disability Discrimination Act
Information Line**
Tel: 0345 622633
Fax: 0345 622644
Website: www.disability.gov.uk/dda

Disability Equipment Register
4 Chatterton Road
Yate
Bristol BS37 4BJ
Tel: 01454 318818
Fax: 01454 883870
Website: www.disabreg.dial.pipex.com
*Nationwide service, via
magazine, to buy and sell used
equipment for people with
disability.*

Disability Law Service
39–45 Cavell Street
London E1 2BP
Tel: 020 7791 9800
Fax: 020 7791 9802
*Provides free legal advice for
people with disabilities.*

**Disability Now (Campaigning
newspaper)**
Editorial Department
6 Market Road
London N7 9PW
Tel: 020 7619 7323
Fax: 020 7619 7331
Minicom: 020 7619 7332
Website: www.disabilitynow.org.uk
*Newspaper publishing news and
views for and about people with
disabilities. Available nation-
wide via newsagents and by
subscription.*

Disability Rights Commission
Tel: 08457 622633
Website: www.drc-gb.org
*An independent body established
to eliminate discrimination
against disabled people and
secure equal opportunities.
Helpline service on all disability
issues, and legal advice with
appropriate support.*

Disability Sport England
Unit 4G, N17 Studios
784–788 High Road
Tottenham
London N17 ODA
Tel: 020 8801 4466
Fax: 020 8801 6644
Website: www.disabilitysport.org.uk
*Provides opportunities for
people of all ages with
disabilities to take part in sport.
Has regional offices.*

Disabled Access to Technology Association
Neville House
Neville Road
Bradford BD4 8TU
Tel: 01274 370019
Fax: 01274 723861
Website: www.databradford.org
Trains people with disabilities to enable them to get back to work.

Disabled Christians Fellowship
Global House
Ashley Avenue
Epsom KT18 5AD
Tel: 01372 737046
Fax: 01372 737040
Website: www.throughtheroof.org
Fellowship by correspondence, cassettes, local branches, holidays, youth section, local workshop and day centre.

Disabled Drivers Association
Ashwellthorpe
Norwich NR16 1EX
Tel: 01508 489449
Fax: 01508 488173
Website: www.dda.org.uk
Self-help association offering information and advice and aiming for independence through mobility.

Disabled Drivers Motor Club
Cottingham Way
Thrapston
Northants NN14 4PL
Tel: 01832 734724
Fax: 01832 733816
Website: www.ddmc.org.uk
Offers information service to disabled drivers about ferries, airports and insurance. Subscription for bi-monthly magazine.

Disabled Living Centres Council
Redbank House
4 St Chads Street
Cheetham
Manchester M8 8QA
Tel: 0161 834 1044
Fax: 0161 839 0802
Textphone: 0161 839 0885
Website: www.dlcc.org.uk
Coordinates work of Disabled Living Centres UK wide. Offers lists of centres and the different services that they provide.

Disabled Living Foundation
380–384 Harrow Road
London W9 2HU
Helpline: 0845 130 9177
Tel: 020 7289 6111
Fax: 020 7266 2922
Minicom: 020 7432 8009
Website: www.dlf.org.uk
Provides information on all kinds of equipment for people with special needs.

Disabled Motorists Federation
Unit B1
Greenwood Court
Cartmel Drive
Shrewsbury SY1 3TB
Tel: 01743 463072
Self-help organization offering
information to drivers with
disabilities and campaigning on
their behalf for better motoring
and public transport facilities.
Arranges concessions for ferry
bookings. Local groups.

**Disablement Income Group
(DIG)**
PO Box 5743
Finchingfield
Braintree CM7 4PW
Tel: 01371 811621
Fax: 01371 811633
Promotes the financial welfare of
disabled people with advice
service on rights and benefits.

**Disablement Income Group
Scotland**
5 Quayside Street
Edinburgh EH6 6EJ
Tel: 0131 555 2811
Fax: 0131 554 7076
Offers information and advice
on welfare benefits to disabled
people and their carers in
Scotland.

**Driver and Vehicle Licensing
Authority (DVLA)**
Medical Branch
Longview Road
Morriston
Swansea SA99 1TU
Helpline: 0870 600 0301
Tel: 0870 240 0009
Fax: 01792 783779/761100
Website: www.dvla.gov.uk
Information and advice for
motorists with disabilities.

**Employment Opportunities
for People with Disabilities**
123 Minories
London EC3N 1NT
Tel: 020 7481 2727
Fax: 020 7481 9797
Website: www.opportunities.org.uk
Helps people with disabilities
find and retain employment
through training, mock inter-
views, assessment, graduate
scheme and support during
placements. Regional centres
offer training on disability
awareness to employers.

English Heritage
Customer Services Department
PO Box 569
Swindon SN2 2YP
Tel: 01793 414910
Fax: 01793 414926
Website: english-heritage.org.uk
Offers information on suitable
sites, available aids, access and
parking.

**Equal Opportunities
Commission**
Arndale House
Arndale Centre
Manchester M4 3EQ
Tel: 0845 601 5901
Fax: 0161 838 1733
Website: www.eoc.org.uk
*Investigates cases of sex
discrimination and equal pay
issues. Offers a range of
information, freely available on
the website.*

Family Fund Trust
PO Box 50
York YO1 9ZX
Helpline: 0845 130 4542
Tel: 01904 621115
Fax: 01904 652625
Website: www.familyfundtrust.org.uk
*Offers information and grants
for items such as bedding,
holidays or driving lessons to
families in the UK with children
of up to 16 years with special
care needs.*

Family Service Units
207 Old Marylebone Road
London NW1 5QP
Tel: 020 7402 5175
Fax: 020 7724 1829
Website: www.fsu.org.uk
*Offers a range of support to
children and families
disadvantaged by poverty and at
risk of social exclusion.*

Family Welfare Association
501–505 Kingsland Road
London E8 4AU
Tel: 020 7254 6251
Fax: 020 7249 5443
Website: www.fwa.org.uk
*Runs family drop-in centres and
mental health residential homes.
Education and welfare grants
available. Only accept referrals
in writing from professionals.*

**Gardening for the Disabled
Trust**
The Freight
Cranbrook TN17 3PG
Tel: 01580 712196
Website:
www.gardeningintheweald.co.uk
*Offers practical advice and
information to help keen
gardeners keep gardening,
despite disability or age. Also
offers small grants.*

General Osteopathic Council
Osteopathy House
176 Tower Bridge Road
London SE1 3LU
Tel: 020 7357 6655
Fax: 020 7357 0011
Website: www.osteopathy.org.uk
*Regulatory body that offers
information to the public and
lists of accredited osteopaths.*

Gingerbread (Organization for Lone Parent Families)
7 Sovereign Court
Sovereign Close
London E1W 3HW
Helpline: 0800 018 4318
Tel: 020 7488 9300
Fax: 020 7488 9333
Website: www.gingerbread.org.uk
National network of self-help groups for lone parents and children. Has publications and advice line covering legal, benefits and emotional issues.

Help for Health Trust
Highcroft
Romsey Road
Winchester SO22 5DH
Tel: 01962 849100
Website: www.hfht.org
Monitors the quality of service provided by NHS Direct.

Holiday Care
2nd Floor Imperial Buildings
Victoria Road
Horley RH6 7PZ
Tel: 01293 774535
Fax: 01293 784647
Website: www.holidaycare.org.uk
Provides holiday advice on venues and tour operators for people with special needs.

Holiday Homes Trust (Scouts)
Gilwell Park
Bury Road
Chingford E4 7QW
Tel: 020 8433 7290
Fax: 020 8433 7184
Website:
www.scoutbase.org.uk/hq-info
Offers low-cost, self-catering holidays on fully commercial holiday parks for disabled and disadvantaged people. No scouting connection necessary.

Home Care Support
382 Hillcross Avenue
Morden SM4 4EX
Tel: 020 8542 0348
Fax: 020 8542 0348
Private agency providing personal care in the home. Available 24 hours a day.

Incontact
United House
North Road
London N7 9DP
Tel: 0870 770 3246
Fax: 0870 770 3249
Website: www.incontact.org
Incontact is a national charity for people affected by bladder and bowel problems, providing support and information and representing the interests of people with continence problems.

**Independent Living
Alternatives**
Trafalgar House
Grenville Place
London NW7 3SA
Tel: 020 8906 9265
Fax: 020 8906 9265
Website: www.i-l-a.fsnet.co.uk
*Gives advice on how to obtain
cash entitlement from benefit
agencies by direct payment in
lieu of meals on wheels or home
help from local authorities.*

Independent Living Fund
PO Box 183
Nottingham NG8 3RD
Tel: 0115 942 8191
Fax: 0115 929 3156
Website: www.ilf.org.uk
*Offers financial assistance in the
UK for buying personal and/or
domestic care. Referral via
Social Services.*

**Institute for Complementary
Medicine**
PO Box 194
London SE16 7QZ
Tel: 020 7237 5165
Fax: 020 7237 5175
Website: www.icmedicine.co.uk
*Umbrella group for
complementary medicine
organizations. Offers informed,
safe choice to public, British
register of practitioners and
refers to accredited training
courses.*

John Grooms
50 Scrutton Street
London EC2A 4PH
Tel: 020 7452 2000
Fax: 020 7452 2001
Website: www.johngrooms.org.uk
*Charity providing a range of
residential care, housing,
holidays and work across the
UK.*

Keep Able Ltd
Sterling Park
Pedmore Road
Brierley Hill DY5 1TB
Tel: 01384 484544
Fax: 01384 480802
Website: www.keepable.co.uk
*Distributors of equipment and
aids for the elderly and less able.
Home assessments for stairlifts,
wheelchairs etc. Available via
mail order. Some regional
stores.*

Law Centres Federation
Duchess House
18–19 Warren Street
London W1T 5LR
Tel: 020 7387 8570
Fax: 020 7387 8368
Website: www.lawcentres.org.uk
*Headquarters of national law
centres. Can refer to local law
centres and website for free
information and advice.*

Law Society
114 Chancery Lane
London WC2A 1PL
Tel: 020 7320 5793
Fax: 020 7831 0170
Website: www.gsdnet.org.uk
*Offers help and support to law
students and solicitors with
disabilities.*

Leonard Cheshire
30 Millbank
London SW1P 4QD
Tel: 020 7802 8200
Fax: 020 7802 8250
Website: www.leonard-cheshire.org
*Offers care, support and a wide
range of information for
disabled people between 18 and
65 years in the UK and
worldwide. Respite and
residential homes, holidays and
rehabilitation.*

**Liberty (The National Council
for Civil Liberties)**
21 Tabard Street
London SE1 4LA
Helpline: 020 7378 8659
Tel: 020 7403 3888
Fax: 020 7407 5354
Website: www.yourrights.org.uk
*Pressure group which protects
and extends human rights and
civil liberties. Offers information
and free legal advice helpline.*

Listening Books
12 Lant Street
London SE1 1QH
Tel: 020 7407 9417
Fax: 020 7403 1377
Website: www.listening-books.org.uk
*Offers talking books on tape for
adults and children suitable for
anyone who cannot read in the
usual way. Subscription for
lending library of tapes by mail
order.*

The Lodge
Regional Rehabilitation Centre
Hunters Road
Newcastle upon Tyne NE2 4NR
Tel: 01912 195640
Fax: 01912 195647
*NHS communication aid centre
for people with disabilities.
Open referral.*

**Long-Term Medical Conditions
Alliance (LMCA)**
c/o Unit 212
16 Baldwins Gardens
London EC1N 7RJ
Tel: 020 7813 3637
Fax: 020 7813 3640
Website: www.lmca.org.uk
*Campaigns to improve the
quality of life of people with
long-term medical conditions.*

Low Pay Unit
10 Dukes Road
London WC1H 9AD
Helpline: 020 7431 7385
Tel: 020 7435 4268
Website: www.lowpayunit.org.uk
Offers information leaflets and
telephone advice on employment
rights.

Medic-Alert Foundation
1 Bridge Wharf
156 Caledonian Road
London N1 9UU
Helpline: 0800 581420
Tel: 020 7833 3034
Fax: 020 7713 5653
Website: www.medicalert.org.uk
A body-worn identification system
for people with hidden medical
conditions. 24-hour emergency
telephone number. Offers selection
of jewellery with internationally
recognized medical symbol.

Mobility Advice and Vehicle
Information Service (MAVIS)
O Wing, Macadam Avenue
Old Wokingham Road
Crowthorne RG45 6XD
Tel: 01344 661000
Fax: 01344 661066
Website: www.mobility-unit.dft.gov.uk
Government department offering
driving and vehicle assessment
to people with disabilities.

Mobility Information Service
and Disabled Motorists Club
National Mobility Centre
Unit B1 Greenwood Court
Cartmel Drive
Shrewsbury SY1 3TB
Tel: 01743 463072
Fax: 01743 463065
Website: www.mis.org.uk
Information on mobility.
Driving assessment for disabled
drivers at regional centres.

Motability
Goodman House
Station Approach
Harlow CM20 2ET
Tel: 01279 635666
Fax: 01279 632000
Website: www.motability.co.uk
Advises people with disabilities
about powered wheelchairs,
scooters, new and used cars, how
to adapt them to their needs and
obtain funding via the
Disability Living Allowance.

**National Centre for
Independent Living**
250 Kennington Lane
London SE11 5RD
Tel: 020 7587 1663
Fax: 020 7582 2469
Website: www.ncil.org.uk
*Provides information,
consultancy and training on
personal assistance and direct
payments. Advice for obtaining
payment from the benefits
system to enable people to buy
private personal care instead of
receiving it via the local
authority.*

**National Council for Hospice
and Specialist Palliative Care**
1st Floor, 34–44 Britannia Street
London WC1X 9JG
Helpline: 0870 903 3903
Tel: 020 7520 8299
Fax: 020 7520 8298
Website:
www.hospice-spc-council.org.uk
*Umbrella organization, which
promotes and extends palliative
care system.*

**National Disabled Persons
Housing Service (HODIS)**
17 Priory Street
York YO1 6ET
Tel: 01904 653888
Fax: 01904 653 999
Website: www.hodis.org.uk
*Promotes and supports the
creation of local housing services
for people with disabilities.*

National Gardens Scheme
Hatchlands Park
East Clandon
Guildford GU4 7RT
Tel: 01483 211535
Fax: 01483 211537
Website: www.ngs.org.uk
*Provides list of privately owned
gardens which, for a donation to
charity, are open to the public at
certain times of year.*

**National Institute of Medical
Herbalists**
56 Longbrook Street
Exeter EX4 6AH
Tel: 01392 426022
Fax: 01392 498963
Website: www.nimh.org.uk
*Professional body representing
qualified, practising medical
herbalists. Offers lists of
accredited medical herbalists.*

National Trust Membership Department
36 Queen Anne's Gate
London SW1H 9AS
Tel: 0870 609 5380
Fax: 020 7222 5097
Website: www.nationaltrust.org.uk

Open University (OU)
Disability Advisory Services
Walton Hall
Milton Keynes MK7 6AA
Tel: 01908 652255
Fax: 01908 659956
Website: www.open.ac.uk
Offers advice to people who wish to study accredited educational courses at home.

Patients Association
PO Box 935
Harrow HA1 3YJ
Helpline: 0845 608 4455
Tel: 020 8423 9111
Fax: 020 8423 9119
Website:
www.patients-association.com
Provides advice on patients' rights. Leaflets and self-help directory available.

Pensions Advisory Service (OPAS)
11 Belgrave Road
London SW1V 1RB
Tel: 020 7233 8080
Fax: 020 7233 8016
Website: www.opas.org.uk
Free help to people with problems with occupational, personal and stakeholder pensions. State pensions are not dealt with but referred appropriately.

Possum Controls Ltd
8 Farmbrough Close
Stocklake Industrial Estate
Aylesbury HP20 1DQ
Tel: 01296 461000
Fax: 01296 461001
Website: www.possum.co.uk
Manufacturers of communication aids and other equipment to the NHS. Repair service available. Self-referral.

Prentke Romich International (PRI) Ltd
Minerva House
Minerva Business Park
Lynch Wood
Peterborough PE2 6FT
Tel: 01733 370470
Fax: 01733 391939
Website: www.prentromint.com
Sells communications aids and accessories. Repair service.

Princess Royal Trust for Carers
30 George Street
Glasgow G2 1LH
Tel: 0141 221 5066
Fax: 0141 221 4623
and
142 Minories
London EC3N 1LB
Tel: 020 7480 7788
Fax: 020 7481 4729
Website: www.carers.org
Trust formed to provide information, support and practical help with carer centres.

Queen Elizabeth Foundation for Disabled People
Leatherhead Court
Woodlands Road
Leatherhead KT22 0BN
Tel: 01372 841100
Fax: 01372 844072
Website: www.qefd.org
Provides information, demonstrations, assessment and training on outdoor mobility for professionals and people with disabilities.

RADAR (Royal Assoc. for Disability and Rehabilitation)
12 City Forum
250 City Road
London EC1V 8AF
Tel: 020 7250 3222
Fax: 020 7250 0212
Minicom 020 7250 4119
Website: www.radar.org.uk

Campaigns to improve rights and care of disabled people. Offers advice on every aspect of living with a disability and refers to other agencies for training and rehabilitation.

Rail Unit for Disabled Passengers Switchboard
Helpline: 08700 005 151
Queries about travelling within the UK rail network referred to appropriate areas for advice. Enquirers must provide specific details of destination in order to be referred to appropriate railway company.

Relate (Marriage Guidance)
Herbert Gray College
Little Church Street
Rugby CV21 3AP
Helpline: 0845 130 4010
Tel: 01788 573241
Fax: 01788 535007
Website: www.relate.org.uk
Offers relationship counselling via local branches. Publications from Relate bookshop, mail order; health, sexual, self-esteem, depression,bereavement, remarriage issues.

REMAP
National Organizer
Hazeldene
Ightham
Sevenoaks TN15 9AD
Tel: 0845 1300 456
Fax: 0845 1300 789
Website: www.remap.org.uk
Makes or adapts aids, when not
commercially available, for
people with disabilities at no
charge to the disabled person.
Local branches.

Research Council for
Complementary Medicine
27A Devonshire Street
London W1G 6PN
Tel: 020 7935 7499
Website: www.rccm.org.uk
Enables research and provides
information on existing
research. Has data base of
research which can be accessed
via website.

Royal Horticultural Society
80 Vincent Square
London SW1P 2PE
Tel: 020 7834 4333
Fax: 020 7821 3020
Website: www.rhs.org.uk
Offers information on disabled
access/wheelchair availability at
gardens linked to the RHS.

Scottish Association of Health
Councils
24A Palmerston Place
Edinburgh EH12 5AL
Tel: 0131 220 4101
Fax: 0131 220 4108
Website: www.show.scot.nhs.uk/sahc

Sequal Trust
3 Ploughmans Corner
Wharf Road
Ellesmere SY12 0EJ
Tel: 01691 624222
Fax: 01691 624222
Website: www.the-sequal-trust.org.uk
Fundraising charity which helps
provide communication aids for
people disabled with speech,
movement or learning
difficulties.

Shaftesbury Society
16 Kingston Road
London SW19 1JZ
Tel: 020 8239 5555
Fax: 020 8239 5580
Website: www.shaftesburysoc.org.uk
Christian organization provides
residential centres, schools,
colleges and holiday centres for
disabled people of all religious
faiths. Has prayer line.

Shirley Price Aromatherapy
Essentia House
Upper Bond Street
Hinckley LE10 1RS
Tel: 01455 615466
Fax: 01455 615054
Website: www.shirleyprice.com
*Sources and supplies natural
pure essential oils and carriers
for aromatherapy. International
college training to professional
standards and lists of local
therapists accredited by ISPA
(International Society of
Professional Aromatherapists).
Mail order.*

**SPOD (Association to aid the
Sexual and Personal
Relationships of People with a
Disability)**
286 Camden Road
London N7 0BJ
Helpline: 020 7607 9191
Tel: 020 7607 8851
Fax: 020 7700 0236
Website: www.spod-uk.org
*Provides information and
advice on the problems in sex
and personal relationships,
which disability can cause.*

Sunrise Medical
Tel: 01384 446688
Fax: 01384 446699
Website: www.sunrisemedical.co.uk

**Talking Newspapers
Association UK**
National Recording Centre
Browning Road
Heathfield TN21 8DB
Tel: 01435 866102
Fax: 01435 865422
Website: www.tnauk.org.uk
*Lists 200 national newspapers
and magazines on tape,
computer, CD-ROM and email
for loan to visually impaired,
blind and physically disabled
people. Annual subscription.*

Telework Association
WREN Telecottage
Stoneleigh Park
Kenilworth CV8 2RR
Helpline: 0800 616008
Tel: 02476 696986
Fax: 02476 696538
Website: www.telework.org.uk
*Information handbook on legal
and practical aspects of setting
up home business.*

THRIVE
Sir Geoffrey Udall Centre
Beech Hill
Reading RG7 2AT
Tel: 0118 988 5688
Fax: 0118 988 5677
Website: www.thrive.org.uk
Information on gardening and horticulture for training, employment, therapy and health. Uses gardening to help disabled and disadvantaged elderly people to have a better quality of life.

Ulverscroft Large Print Books
FA Thorpe Publishing Ltd
The Green
Bradgate Road
Anstey LE7 7FU
Tel: 0116 236 4325
Fax: 0116 234 0205
Website: www.ulverscroft.co.uk
Publishes large print books which are available at libraries and via mail order.

J D Williams (Special Collection)
Freepost
PO Box 123
Manchester M99 1BN
Tel: 0161 237 1200
Fax: 0161 238 2626
Website: www.specialcollection.com
A mail order catalogue of fashion clothing and footwear available in large sizes.

Winged Fellowship Trust
Angel House
20/32 Pentonville Road
London N1 9XD
Tel: 020 7833 2594
Fax: 020 7278 0370
Website: www.wft.org.uk
Provides holidays at their own UK centres and respite care for people with severe physical disabilities by providing volunteer carers. Also arranges holidays for people with dementia/Alzheimer's disease and their own carers.

Yoga for Health Foundation
Ickwell Bury
Biggleswade SG18 9EF
Tel: 01767 627271
Fax: 01767 627266
Website:
www.yogaforhealthfoundation.co.uk
Teacher training for remedial yoga.

Communication Aids Centres

Access to Communication and Technology
Oak Tree Lane Centre
91 Oak Tree Lane
Selly Oak
Birmingham B29 6JA
Tel: 0121 627 8235
Fax: 0121 627 8892
Website: http://www.bscht.org.uk/
Services/rehab/fraRehab2.htm
Advice on communications aids. Open referral.

ACS (Assistive Communication Service)
2nd Floor, North Wing
Charing Cross Hospital
Fulham Palace Road
London W6 8RF
Tel: 020 8846 1057
Fax: 020 8846 7610
Offers assessment, advice and recommendation for people needing communications aid system. Open referral.

Bristol CAC (Communication Aid Centre)
Speech Therapy and Language Department
Frenchay Hospital
Frenchay
Bristol BS16 1LE
Tel: 0117 975 3946
Fax: 0117 918 6558
Website: www.cacfrenchay.nhs.uk
NHS communication aid centre offering assessment, advice and recommendation for people with disabilities. Training and research. Open referral.

CAC (Communication Aid Centre)
Musgrave Park Hospital
Stockmans Lane
Belfast BT9 7JB
Tel: 02890 669501
Fax: 02890 683662
NHS centre providing assessment and advice on communication aids for people with disabilities. NHS referral only.

Cambridge Adaptive Communications
8 Farnborough Close
Stocklake
Aylesbuiry HP20 1DQ
Tel: 01296 461002
Fax: 01296 461107
Website: www.cameleon-web.com
Provide products, tools, services and assessment to aid verbal and non-verbal communication and improve computer accessibility. Have repair service.

Cardiff CAC (Communication Aid Centre)
ALAC, Artificial Limb and Appliances Service
Rookwood Hospital
Fairwater Road
Llandaff
Cardiff CF5 2YN
Tel: 02920 313956
Fax: 02920 555156
NHS centre providing artificial limbs, appliances and communications aids to people with disabilities. Open referral.

Keycomm-Lothian Communication Technology Service
St Giles Centre
40 Broomhouse Crescent
Edinburgh EH11 3UB
Tel: 0131 443 6775
Fax: 0131 443 5121
Communication aids centre for Lothian regions working with health, education and social needs. Caters for children and adults with severe communication impairment and offers assessment, training and has loan bank of equipment. Open referral.

Scottish Centre of Technology for the Communication Impaired (SCTCI, WESTMARC)
Southern General Hospital
1345 Govan Road
Glasgow G51 4TF
Tel: 0141 201 2619
Fax: 0141 201 2618
NHS centre offering assessment and advice to people with disabilities. Open referral.

Index

Have you found **Motor Neurone Disease – the 'at your fingertips'**
guide practical and useful? If so, you may be interested in other
books from Class Publishing.

Beating Depression – the 'at your fingertips' guide
NEW TITLE £14.99

Dr Stefan Cembrowicz
and Dr Dorcas Kingham
This positive handbook, written by
two medical experts, gives practical
advice on overcoming depression
and anxiety. It covers the different
treatments available, and offers self-
help techniques.

'A sympathetic and understanding guide.'
Marjorie Wallace, Chief Executive, SANE

Parkinson's – the 'at your fingertips' guide
SECOND EDITION £14.99

Dr Marie Oxtoby
and Professor Adrian Williams
If you have any questions about
managing Parkinson's, about
medication and treatment, about
benefits and finance, about transport
and holidays, and about where to
turn to for help and support – you will
find the answers here.

'This book provides the answers to so
many questions.'
Mary G Baker MBE, Former Chief
Executive, Parkinson's Disease Society

Multiple Sclerosis – the 'at your fingertips' guide
£14.99

Professor Ian Robinson, Dr Stuart
Neilson and Dr Frank Clifford Rose
Straightforward and positive answers
to all your questions about MS, with
over 200 real questions included
from people with MS and their
families. Armed with this book, you
will feel able to cope with the
challenges that MS presents, to live
a full and active life.

'An invaluable resource.'
Jan Hatch, MS Society

Positive Action for Health and Wellbeing – the complete programme
NEW TITLE £29.99

Dr Brian Roet
Dr Roet explains simply and clearly
about the positive steps you can take
to promote your own health and
wellbeing. Includes a practical guide,
a personal progress diary and a
double cassette pack.

'Over the years I have read countless
self-help books and none helped. No
other book has ever had this effort on
me.'
S.G. Hampshire

Dementia: Alzheimer's and other dementias – the 'at your fingertips' guide
SECOND EDITION £14.99

Harry Cayton, Dr Nori Graham
and Dr James Warner
At last – a book that tells you
everything you need to know about
Alzheimer's and other dementias.

'An invaluable contribution to
understanding all forms of dementia.'
Dr Jonathan Miller CBE, President of the
Alzheimer's Disease Society

Sexual Health for Men – the 'at your fingertips' guide
NEW TITLE £14.99

Dr Philip Kell and Vanessa Griffiths
This practical handbook answers
hundreds of real questions from men
with erectile dysfunction and their
partners. Up to 50% of the
population aged over 60 is impotent
– though they need not be, if they
take appropriate action.

PRIORITY ORDER FORM

Cut out or photocopy this form and send it (post free in the UK) to:

Class Publishing Priority Service   **Tel: 01752 202 301**
FREEPOST (PAM 6210)
Plymouth PL6 7ZZ

                               Fax: 01752 202 333

	Please send me urgently (*tick boxes below*)	*Post included* *price per copy (UK only)*
☐	**Motor Neurone Disease – the 'at your fingertips' guide** (ISBN 1 85959 047 0)	£17.99
☐	**Beating Depression – the 'at your fingertips' guide** (ISBN 1 85959 063 2)	£17.99
☐	**Parkinson's – the 'at your fingertips' guide** (ISBN 1 872362 96 6)	£17.99
☐	**Multiple Sclerosis – the 'at your fingertips' guide** (ISBN 1 872362 94 X)	£17.99
☐	**Positive Action for Health and Wellbeing – the complete programme** (ISBN 1 85959 041 1)	£32.99
☐	**Dementia: Alzheimer's and other dementias – the 'at your fingertips' guide** (ISBN 1 85959 075 6)	£17.99
☐	**Sexual Health for Men – the 'at your fingertips' guide** (ISBN 1 85959 011 X)	£17.99

TOTAL _____

Easy ways to pay

Cheque: I enclose a cheque payable to Class Publishing for £ _____

Credit card: Please debit my

☐ Mastercard   ☐ Visa   ☐ Amex   ☐ Switch

Number _____ Expiry date _____

Name _____

My address for delivery is _____

_____

Town _____ County _____ Postcode _____

Telephone number (*in case of query*) _____

Credit card billing address if different from above _____

_____

Town _____ County _____ Postcode _____